Birth After Caesarean

Your Journey to a Better Birth

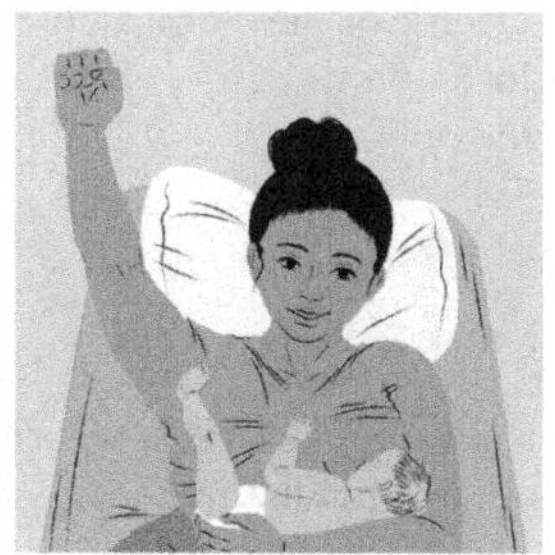

Hazel Keedle, PhD

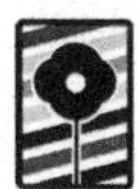

Praeclarus Press, LLC

---

www.PraeclarusPress.com

Praeclarus Press, LLC
2504 Sweetgum Lane
Amarillo, Texas 79124 USA
806-367-9950
www.PraeclarusPress.com

DISCLAIMER

The information contained in this publication is advisory only and is not intended to replace sound clinical judgment or individualized patient care. The author disclaims all warranties, whether expressed or implied, including any warranty as the quality, accuracy, safety, or suitability of this information for any particular purpose.

ISBN: 978-1-946665-58-4

Cover Design: Ken Tackett
Developmental Editing: Kathleen Kendall-Tackett
Copyediting: Chris Tackett
Layout & Design: Nelly Murariu

Acknowledgements

I would like to thank the many individuals that have helped this book happen. Firstly, the women who have been interviewed, recorded their experiences, piloted, and taken part in the VBAC in Australia surveys. Your willingness to share your experiences are the basis of my research and I am truly grateful. I am also so thankful to the women who shared their stories for this book; their generosity, honesty, and enthusiasm make this book relatable to all who will read it.

Thank you to my friends and colleagues who have encouraged and at times, read sections of the book for me. Thank you, Catherine Bell, for writing a section on Birth Mapping for the book. Thank you, Pixie, for your poetry and friendship; it has been so important to me. Thank you to my PhD supervisors and now friends Professor Hannah Dahlen, Associate Professor Elaine Burns, and Professor Virginia Schmied. Your faith and support encouraged me to conduct and love research.

To my family, my mum who supports me from across the oceans, my brother, my uncles, and my cousins who remind me how proud my dad and granny would be. My husband Warren; he is my biggest supporter, best friend and partner, and has stamped on any self-doubt I have voiced. I love you more!

Finally, I want to thank my children, Freyja and Perran. They have been patient while I wrote, and they have remained excited throughout. They inspire me and their births are the reasons this book was written.

TABLE OF CONTENTS

Glossary of terms ix

Chapter 1 The Journey to VBAC 1

My Journey to VBAC 2

My Research Journey 5

My PhD Journey 5

Phase 1 6

Phase 2 6

Phase 3 7

Book Summary 8

Language 8

Chapter 2 Your Previous Caesarean 13

Birth Trauma 13

Birth Trauma Experiences 14

Symptoms of Birth Trauma 16

Seeking Help 17

Debriefing 18

Accessing Debriefing 20

Summary 20

Chapter 3 Your Birth Options 21

Options 21

Risks of VBAC 24

Uterine Rupture 24

Identifying a Uterine Rupture 26

Following a Uterine Rupture 27

Risks of Elective/Emergency Caesarean 28
Long-Term Complications 29
VBAC Rates 31
Length of Time Between Caesarean and the Next Birth 32
VBAC Calculators 33
Summary 35

Chapter 4 Can I Have a VBAC if...? 37
"I Have a Higher BMI" 37
"I Need to Be Induced" 38
"I Have Gestational Diabetes Mellitus (GDM)" 40
"My Baby is Breech" 41
"I Am Pregnant with Twins" 43
"I've Had More than One Caesarean" 43
"I Have a Special Scar" 45
"I Choose to Birth at Home or in a Birth Centre" 48
Summary 49

Chapter 5 Having Control 51
Introduction 51
Feminism and Birth 52
The First Wave 52
The Second Wave 54
Third Wave 57
Reproductive Justice 58
Birth Plans 62
Birth Mapping for Birth after Caesarean – Catherine Bell 63
The Three Scenarios Exercise 67
Three Scenario Examples 70
Summary 72

Chapter 6 Having Confidence **73**

Why is Confidence Important? 73

How Can I Gain Confidence in My Body? 75

Preparing Your Body 75

Yoga 77

Increasing Knowledge: Alternative Birthing Classes 79

Peer Support 81

Podcasts 81

Summary 82

Chapter 7 Having a Relationship **83**

Choose Your Team 83

Different Models of Care 86

Research Around CoC 87

Survey Results for Models of Care 88

Appointment Times 89

Receiving Positive Support 90

Receiving Hurtful Comments from Midwife or Doctor 91

MADM & MORi Scores 91

What is Good Support? 92

How to Find a Coc Model of Care 92

Choosing a Doula 93

Summary 94

Chapter 8 Having an Active Labour **97**

Importance of Active Labour 98

Preparing for Being Active 99

How to Be Active in Labour When Monitored (CTG) 101

Water Immersion and Waterbirth 106

Summary 107

Chapter 9 Planning for a Gentle Caesarean 109
What Does a Gentle Caesarean Look Like? 109
Maternal-Assisted Caesarean 110
Skin to Skin in Theatre 111
Summary 112

Chapter 10 Women's Stories 113
Caroline - VBAC with a Classical Scar 117
Kari – VBAC after a Uterine Rupture 123
Birth History 123
Pregnancy After Rupture 129
Brianna – VBAC 144
1st Baby 144
2nd Baby 144
Hannah – VBAC with GDM 147
Jordon – VBAC 153
Erin – Homebirth after 2 Caesareans 157
The HBA2C Birth of Samara 157
Siobhan – VBAC with ECV for Breech 163
Daniella –VBAC after 3 Caesareans (VBA3C) 171
Birth Story of Artemis Willa – VBA2C 171
Naomi – VBAC with an Inverted T scar 177
Emili – Homebirth after 2 Caesareans 183
Hayley – Breech VBAC 191
Jasmine – VBAC 201
Jemila – VBAC 203
Laura – Healing VBAC with Lotus Birth 208
Sasha – Homebirth after 2 Caesareans 215

Final Thoughts 219

References 221

Glossary of terms

ANTENATAL: The period during pregnancy up to labour

BODY MASS INDEX: A person's weight in kilograms divided by the square of height in meters

BREECH PRESENTATION: When a baby is in a bottom down position instead of a head down position

CTG: Cardiotocography used for continuous fetal monitoring

CONTINUITY OF CARE (COC): The same HCP providing maternity care throughout pregnancy, birth, and postnatal care

ENDOMETRITIS: Inflammation or irritation of the lining of the uterus usually due to infection

FRAGMENTED CARE: Seeing different healthcare providers during pregnancy appointments, labour, birth, and in the postnatal period

HAEMATURIA: The presence of blood in the urine

HEALTHCARE PROVIDERS (HCP): Healthcare providers, which includes midwives and doctors

HOMEBIRTH AFTER CAESAREAN (HBAC): When women plan or have a VBAC at home

INTERDELIVERY INTERVAL: The length of time between the previous caesarean and the next birth

INTERPREGNANCY INTERVAL: The time between the previous caesarean and conception of the next pregnancy

MOTHER'S AUTONOMY IN DECISION MAKING (MADM) SCALE: Measures autonomy in decision-making in maternity care (Vedam et al., 2017a)

MOTHERS ON RESPECT INDEX (MORI): Measures women's experiences of their interactions with HCP (Vedam et al., 2017b)

MIDWIFERY GROUP PRACTICE (MGP): CoC with a midwife working within a group of midwives, can be in a public or private model

NEXT BIRTH AFTER CAESAREAN (NBAC): Used for the option of elective caesarean or VBAC in the next or current pregnancy

POSTNATAL: The period after having a baby

POSTNATAL DEPRESSION: A common, but debilitating condition that affects one in seven women following the birth of their baby. Unlike the baby blues, which passes on its own, postnatal depression can be long-lasting, and affect the ability to cope with a new baby (https://www.cope.org.au/new-parents/postnatal-mental-health-conditions/postnatal-depression/)

POSTPARTUM HAEMORRHAGE: The loss of 500 ml or more of blood from the genital tract within 24 hours of the birth of a baby. PPH can be minor (500–1000 ml) or major (more than 1000 ml)

POSTTRAUMATIC STRESS DISORDER (PTSD): A particular set of reactions that can develop in people who have been through a traumatic event that threatened their life or safety, or that of others around them (https://www.beyondblue.org.au/the-facts/anxiety/types-of-anxiety/ptsd)

PRIVATELY PRACTISING MIDWIFE (PPM): Self-employed midwives who may work independently or in an MGP. Most PPMs offer CoC across the continuum and may provide homebirth services

RANDOMISED CONTROLLED TRIAL (RCT): A trial where subjects are randomly assigned to an experiment group or a control group to compare treatments/interventions

UTERINE RUPTURE: Complete disruption of the uterine muscle and the uterine serosa (Vandenberghe et al., 2019)

VAGINAL BIRTH AFTER CAESAREAN (VBAC): When a woman plans/has a vaginal birth in her next or current pregnancy following at least one previous caesarean. Antenatal – the period of pregnancy and pre-labour

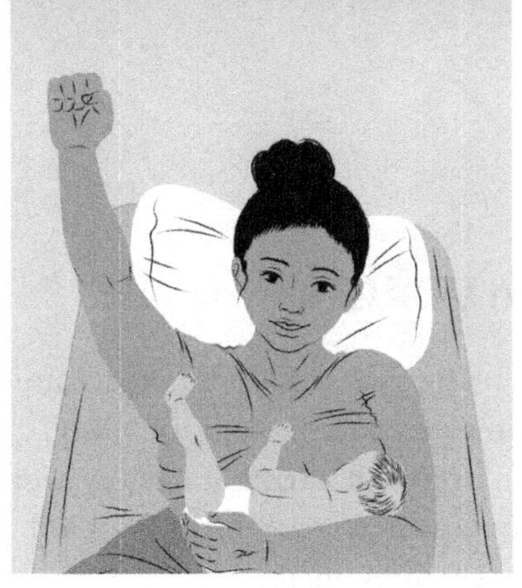

Chapter 1

THE JOURNEY TO VBAC

This book explores your birth options after having a previous caesarean. It is written as a journey. Every journey starts with a beginning. The beginning in this journey is your previous caesarean or caesareans. The journey is your experience of decision-making and planning your next birth, which may start before your next pregnancy but becomes more important and real during your pregnancy. Your hoped-for destination is having the best birthing experience for you. This might be a VBAC, but you may also find yourself at a similar but different destination of a repeat caesarean. This isn't the destination as your birthing experience has many onward ramifications for your experiences as a woman, a mother, and your future birthing experience.

This book will explore this journey using evidence-based research. In the next section, I will share my own VBAC journey and how I became a VBAC researcher. The research I base this journey on is primarily from my PhD into women's experiences of planning a VBAC in Australia, but I will also dive into my VBAC research library, which is burgeoning with thousands of international research articles on the many different aspects of birth after caesarean.

My Journey to VBAC

In my early days of being a midwife, I didn't give much thought to VBAC, I don't recall any time given to the topic of VBAC during my midwifery training, and I don't recount caring for many women who planned a VBAC. I trained in a large tertiary referral hospital, where interventions and caesareans were commonplace.

As a midwife, I planned to birth my first baby in water at home with a privately practising midwife (PPM), but I experienced something different. At 34 weeks, I was unwell and hospitalised with pneumonia, and at 37 weeks, I had a spontaneous rupture of membranes. I was excited about this warm gush of fluid that popped as I was reading a book on my bed, and after letting my midwife know, I quietly laboured during the evening in bed and then in the bath. The following morning, my midwife assessed me, and after a vaginal examination, reported that my baby was breech and said that I should transfer to hospital. I knew what this meant, as I worked at the local hospital and there was a no vaginal breech birth policy. I cried but obediently packed my bag and went off to hospital, where it was confirmed that my compact, little baby was in a frank breech position with his bottom low down and his feet up by his ears. The obstetrician doing the scan exclaimed to my PPM that he was a perfect size and position for a vaginal breech birth but since we don't do that, let's get ready for a caesarean. I sometimes wish I had walked out at that point and found somewhere or someone who would support a vaginal breech birth, but I was in labour and completely disempowered.

After the caesarean, the obstetrician informed me that she had done a vaginal examination in theatres, and I had been 8 cm dilated. I'm not sure how I was meant to feel with that information. I think she was hinting that I had laboured well, but I felt uncomfortable. In time, I realised that there had been an internal vaginal examination without my consent. On top of this, she didn't inform me at the time, that I was 8 cm or give me an opportunity to make an informed decision about my birthing choices. I felt violated and angry by that examination, and I felt helpless in my ability to have the birth that I had wanted.

I struggled physically after my caesarean. A week later, I was feeling extremely unwell with rigours and pain, and was admitted to hospital with endometritis, which was more commonly known throughout history as "childbed fever." I needed a whole heap of antibiotics and another week in hospital, and although my baby could stay with me, it was challenging caring and feeding him with all the intravenous drips and small hospital bed.

Psychologically, I had a difficult time postnatally. I remember waking up to feed him and feeling that I didn't know if he was really mine. It seems a strange thing to think but the birthing process had been so out of my control, that it seemed a rational thought. I did love being a mum to this little baby boy, though. I loved having him wrapped to me, I loved breastfeeding him, and I loved seeing him grow, but something wasn't right. I would try and ignore the sad feelings or the feelings that I had failed to speak up. I tried to ignore the whole hospital experience.

When my baby was only about 6 months old, I started getting sore nipples and in time, I did a pregnancy test. I was pregnant. I didn't expect this, as I had been fully breastfeeding my baby day and night and I had no return to my menstrual cycle that I was aware of. A scan showed that I was already a few months pregnant and had conceived only 4 months after my caesarean. This sent me into a tailspin, as I was forced to confront a big issue. How was I going to birth this baby? I was also concerned that, feeling as low as I was, there was no way I could cope with two babies and the full house we had with being a full-time stepmum to 3 children under the age of 10.

The PPM from my previous pregnancy had advised I read a book called *The Silent Knife*. This book by Nancy Cohen and Lois Estner in 1983 explored the history and rise of caesareans in the U. S. and challenged the fear around VBAC. I devoured this book and then went online to read recent research about VBAC, and specifically, uterine rupture rates with a short timeframe between the caesarean and planned VBAC. I will discuss this topic in more detail in Chapter 3. I found that the uterine rupture rate was nearly 3%, which was higher than less than 1% for longer times between births. This freaked me out a bit, and I explained with dismay to my husband that I can't have a VBAC. He turned it around and said that a 97% chance of not having a uterine rupture were great stats, and we take greater risks travelling in cars every day. I soaked up that positivity and became determined to have a VBAC.

If only my decision-making and determination was enough for the maternity system to support and encourage my VBAC plans. Being a midwife meant I knew how to navigate the maternity system, but I felt it better to avoid the system altogether. I had to go back to working shifts to be able to access paid maternity leave again, and I would get my kind midwifery colleagues to do my blood pressure and listen to the baby's heart rate. I avoided the potential battle with doctors by not engaging or booking in with a hospital. I missed out on continuity of care, as there were no PPM's working in my area and I didn't seek further afield, as I had a bit of a trust issue after my previous experience.

I planned to have a homebirth after caesarean with a good friend I knew well, who was a midwife and doula. I didn't prepare other than having a beautiful mother blessing. I didn't go through my fears with anyone; I just stuck my head in the sand and was a busy, shift-working mum.

I went into early labour in the early hours of a Saturday morning at 38 weeks. I had a weekend of painful early labour supported by my doula and midwife friend, but the contractions weren't consistent, and the team went home. By Monday morning, I was over it and unfortunately, my team was no longer available. I knew I didn't want to freebirth, so my hubby and I went off to the local tertiary hospital.

I was in active labour once I got there, and the battle began. I was continuously pushed to agree to a caesarean, but I refused. I was told I was too loud and then too quiet, and I had no midwife stay longer than 2 minutes in the room. My hubby managed to get a colleague of mine to travel down and support me, and her timing was perfect. I had a moment of doubt with questions to her regarding my birthing ability. She told me I was strong and that I could do it. That was enough to guide me through transition and I quickly started squatting to push my baby out. At the deadline they had given me as the time they would take me to theatres, I pushed my baby girl out of my vagina. I did it!

I scooped her to my chest and that's where she stayed for skin to skin and her first feed. I was instantly euphoric.

Postnatally, I felt amazing, and I felt healed. I regained trust and belief in my body through birthing her through my vagina. I wondered if other women felt like this.

I was also angry about the lack of support I received during labour, and I wondered how any woman without midwifery knowledge managed to have a VBAC. These questions stayed with me and became a driving force to seek answers. A couple of years later, still with a fire in my belly, I met the inspiring Professor Hannah Dahlen. I had shared my birthing story at a community forum she held, and she approached me. She recommended I do research into this area. In time, I agreed, and Hannah became my principal supervisor and now, she is a dear friend and colleague.

My Research Journey

I started my research journey doing a Master of Nursing (Honours) higher-research degree. I explored women's experiences of planning a homebirth after caesarean. I learnt so much about VBAC from the women I interviewed, and I fell in love with the research process. I wrote a thesis and published my first research paper (Keedle et al., 2015; Keedle, 2015). My enquiring mind was hooked, and I wanted to learn more.

My PhD Journey

I had started my PhD journey even before my master's graduation ceremony; I wasted no time. I was grateful to have the same fantastic supervisor team from my master's and these were Professor Hannah Dahlen, Professor Virginia Schmied, and Dr. Elaine Burns. I am so lucky to have been supervised, guided, and mentored by these amazing women.

For the PhD, I wanted to explore women in all models of maternity care and birth locations. I did a mixed-methods study, which means there was both qualitative and quantitative phases of the study. The title was

"The experiences of women planning a VBAC in Australia." My thesis contained four published academic papers and a book chapter.

Phase 1

The first paper was a qualitative literature review where I found published papers on women's experiences of planning a VBAC, including decision making. During this process, the results were amalgamated in a seven-phase process (called a meta-ethnography) and a new theory was developed (Keedle et al., 2018b).

The theory we (my supervisor team and myself) found was that women go on a journey from pain to power. The pain was the experience of a previous caesarean, and the power was after having a VBAC. The journey had positive peaks and negative troughs, which included becoming knowledgeable and having good support and receiving negative comments. The journey became the thread through the rest of the PhD and is the scaffolding of this book.

Phase 2

The second and third papers explored the qualitative arm of the study (Keedle et al., 2018a; Keedle et al., 2019). I developed an app that enabled women who were pregnant and planning a VBAC to do video or audio recordings about their feelings after appointments with their healthcare provider. I followed 11 women throughout their pregnancies and interviewed them all postnatally. The second paper was a technical paper on the app development and the third paper presented the qualitative data.

The findings from this qualitative arm were that there were four factors that influenced how a woman felt after her birth after caesarean. These factors are control, confidence, relationship, and active labour. If the women felt more in control of their wishes and choices, had more confidence in their birthing ability, had a better relationship with a healthcare provider, and was more active in labour, they felt more resolved and positive after their birthing experience. The opposite was also true. If the women felt they had less control, were less confident, had a poor or no relationship with a specific healthcare provider, and were not encouraged or allowed to be active in labour, then they felt more disappointed and negative about their birthing experience. These four factors are explored in more depth in separate chapters in this book.

Phase 3

The fourth paper in my PhD reported on our Australian National VBAC survey (Keedle et al., 2020). In the survey, we grouped questions on the four different factors and distributed the survey via social media. We had a good response from both women who were currently pregnant and those that had planned a VBAC in the previous 5 years. When analysing the data from the women who had previously planned a VBAC, we found a difference in the results dependent on the model of care the women had. Models of care will be discussed in more details in the relationship chapter.

In this arm of the PhD, we found that women who had continuity of care with a midwife felt more in control, felt more confident, had a relationship with their midwife based on trust and equity, and were more likely to be active during labour and be upright during birth. This was compared to women having continuity with a doctor or having standard maternity care where you see different providers at appointments, during labour and birth, and after having the baby. These results provided interesting information for women choosing a healthcare provider for their birth after caesarean journey and will be discussed in more detail in the relationship chapter.

A fifth paper has also been published which analysed the open-ended text responses in the survey. This paper titled 'From coercion to respectful care: women's interactions with health care providers when planning a VBAC' highlighted the positive and negative interactions women had with health care providers during their pregnancy when planning a VBAC (Keedle et al, 2022).

Book Summary

The chapters in this book will help guide you on your birth after caesarean journey using both the research I have described above and international research. The chapters will flow through your journey. The next chapter will explore your previous caesarean(s). The following chapter will discuss birthing after caesarean options and the evidence behind these options. Then, the four factors will be explored in separate chapters. Following this, there is a chapter full of real women's stories of birth after caesarean. I hope you find the journeys in this book both helpful and illuminating. I hope to provide you with knowledge, hope, and a plan to get the birth that you want.

Language

Just a little note about wording. I am an unashamedly feminist researcher. I have used feminist theories for my master's and PhD. This makes me aware about the impact of language.

I identify as a ciswoman and I am aware that most people who have a previous caesarean identify as women, but you may identify as a transman or nonbinary. If you do, then you are welcome here! I understand that you may have had a difficult previous pregnancy and that may be related to how your body changed during pregnancy, isolation, lack of representation, bullying, and discrimination from healthcare providers (Charter et al., 2018; Garcia-Acosta et al., 2019; Voultsos et al., 2021).

There is a current conversation about the use of inclusive language such as "bodies with uteruses," "people with ovaries," and "people who are pregnant" to rid the assumptions that gender identification depicts the same kind of body or use of that body (Karaian, 2013), and I see the benefits of this. I am also cautious to replace the term woman or women, as to do so could take away the "woman" from the research lens when using a feminist research methodology. By removing the focus on "women," we could lose focus on the reasons those who plan a VBAC can have such a difficult time and why birth trauma exists. During my PhD, I wasn't investigating the nuances and struggles regarding gender discrimination within the medical system, and I believe this should be investigated further in the future. As I address in Chapter 5, the historical and current role of patriarchy and over medicalisation have resulted in women experiencing birth trauma, obstetric violence, and coercion. For trans and nonbinary individuals, there is an extra layer of discrimination.

In this book, I refer to "women" and use she/her pronouns. The reasons for this are reflected in an editorial written in the journal "Women and Birth" by Homer et al. (2020).

> *"However, because women are also marginalized and oppressed in most places around the world, we have chosen not to erase the terms 'woman,' 'mother,' or 'maternity' in our journal. When we use these words, it is not meant to exclude those who give birth and do not identify as women, for whom the honouring principles of respectful maternity care described here are equally important."* (Homer et al., 2020, p. 105)

You may have suffered prejudices in the maternity system due to your identified gender and for that, I am sorry. I believe in feminist inclusivity. I am anti-patriarchy, and pro-people. As Bell Hooks said, "Feminism is for Everybody" (Hooks, 2000).

Throughout maternity and VBAC research, there is a disproportional amount of negative language focused on the woman's body. I will describe them here and then deliberately not use them in this book, as I don't believe the woman's body is faulty. Terms such as "failure to progress," "incompetent cervix," and "failed VBAC" can leave the woman feeling that she (or a body part) is to blame without recognition to the overarching impact of a dysfunctional maternity system.

Terms specific to birth after caesarean include "trial of labour" and "trial of scar," which can be indicative of women being held up in court on a charge of wanting a vaginal birth. The judges of the court have decided that your trial has failed, and you are sentenced to a caesarean. This imagery was described in *Silent Knife* (Cohen & Estner, 1983) and challenged my thoughts on this.

In this book, I will talk about planning an elective caesarean, planning a VBAC, having an elective caesarean, having a VBAC, or having a repeat emergency caesarean. There is no failure. You haven't failed if you choose one birth mode but have another. You are amazing and your choices are valid. Be true to you.

The beginning...

Every journey starts with a beginning
Similar but different destinations
Early days, Caesars seen as commonplace
Were the new norm to all complications

A spontaneous rupture, a warm gush
Of fluid popped, the book I was reading
Wept and obediently packed my bag
Every journey starts with a beginning

My compact little baby bottom down
In breech his feet folded up to his ears
In time, realised birthing choices are
Similar but different destinations

Determined, I soaked up the silent knife
Childbed fever and intravenous drips
Strange thing wrapped to me, was he really mine?
Early days, Caesars seen as commonplace

I avoided a potential battle
By burying my head into the sand
Lost in a tailspin, my sad feelings
Were the new norm to all complications

I started confronting the big issues,
I knew the real battle had begun
Told I was too loud and then too quiet
I firmly refused again and again

For just a moment, I doubted myself
Still my contractions weren't consistent
labored way too early, the team went home
I started confronting the big issues

A doula I knew well, mother blessing
Her timing was perfect, she had told me
That bodies are strong, that I could do it
I knew the real battle had begun

I started squatting close to the deadline
With a fire in my belly, I pushed
My baby out and scooped her to my chest
Told I was too loud and then too quiet

Instantly euphoric, I felt healed
This relationship based on trusting my
Self my amazing body, belief grew
I firmly refused again and again

To doubt or misbelieve in women
Each sailing through their transformations
Hooked through the peaks and the troughs, on a quest
Continuing to flow, to thread through enmeshed

I shared my story at a forum, found
My calling, falling in love with research
my enquiring mind over time never
To doubt or misbelieve in women

Needing answers to all the hard questions
Coming together to share their knowledge
to intertwine the power of their births
Each journeying through their transformations

To embrace VBAC with dignity, strength and self-worth

Pixie Willo, 2021

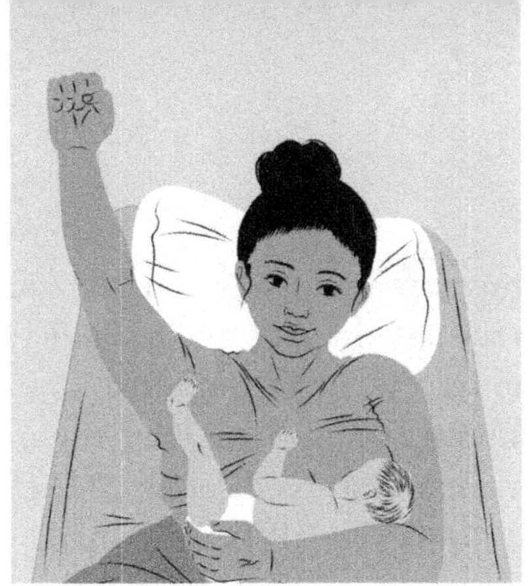

Chapter 2

YOUR PREVIOUS CAESAREAN

I think it is important to start at this point, but I am aware this might be difficult for you to read. Our previous caesareans are often not moments that we want to reflect on. I do feel that through exploring this experience, you may gain some understanding, or at least have some ideas on how you want your next birthing experience to be. So please hold on tight, maybe get some tissues and chocolate nearby, and we will go through this reflection together.

Birth Trauma

In the National VBAC survey, I asked women if they felt their previous caesarean was a traumatic experience and over two thirds of women (69%) stated yes (Keedle et al., 2020). This is a staggering proportion of women who have experienced birth trauma. This leads to questions regarding the definition of birth trauma and the prevalence of birth trauma in the general birthing population.

Much has been written and published on birth trauma. In the survey, I didn't provide a definition on birth trauma to the respondents but relied on the belief that the woman can correctly identify whether she felt the previous caesarean was a traumatic experience or not. This is in line with the definition of "birth trauma lies in the eye of the beholder" (Beck, 2004). The impact of birth trauma is felt by women, partners, fathers, families, and society. Birth trauma can lead to formal diagnosis of posttraumatic stress disorder (PTSD) and/or depression and/or anxiety disorders (Kendall-Tackett, 2014).

Birth Trauma Experiences

Experiences of birth trauma are not only felt by women who have had a previous caesarean, but research suggests they experience higher rates of birth trauma (Keedle et al., 2020). When women are asked to identify the parts of their previous labour and birth that contributed to birth trauma, they identify feelings of losing control, and feeling belittled and unsupported (Baxter, 2020), which can include a lack of informed consent and feeling violated from experiencing obstetric violence (Keedle et al., 2015; Van Der Pijl et al., 2020).

In the paper "The Journey from Pain to Power," the pain was described under the theme "The hurt me" (Keedle et al., 2018b). When women described the feelings during labour, there was often a fear that the life of their baby or themselves was at risk and the language from healthcare providers fuelled the urgency and stress. This quote from a woman in the paper describes her fears:

> *It's like life or death. You don't know if you're going to live or your baby is going to live. You are not told anything. You are just rushed into theatre* (Keedle et al., 2018b, p. 74).

The physical experience of the caesarean also contributed to birth trauma for some women. In the HBAC study, a woman described the impact of her treatment by the healthcare professionals during her caesarean.

> *God, even now it brings up emotions [silence, quiet crying] ... just I mean the experience of having a caesarean so you, you are cut open and then they take the baby and I'm deliriously happy that he's, that he's been born [crying], sorry... but the doctors, but their talking about*

> *their weekend while they are stitching me up, and they are talking about what they are going to do at the weekend, you just feel like a piece of cold meat on the slab, and I remember saying excuse me and asking them a question and it was like it was a big thing* (Jeanne) (Keedle et al., 2015, p. 5).

Another aspect of "the hurt me" theme were the feelings from women that they had failed in having a vaginal birth. These feelings of failure could develop into feelings of self-blame for being ignorant or having a lack of knowledge on how to navigate the challenges of labour.

> *I felt a total sense of failure . . . I felt my body had let me down. It just wasn't the birth I had imagined, and I couldn't get over that* (Keedle et al., 2018b, p. 75).

The way women are treated by healthcare professionals is pivotal in experiences of birth trauma. A recent study explored social media posts on the Dutch "Birth Movement" Facebook page, where women used the tag #genoeggezwegen (known in English as #breakthesilence or #roses-revolution). These 438 deidentified stories were analysed and found many women were disregarded, not taken seriously, felt they were not being heard, not given compassion, and had force used on them, all by healthcare professionals (Van Der Pijl et al., 2020).

> *While I was laying there, in all my naked vulnerability, she barked at me, twice: I should not interfere. With her hand in between my legs, looking me straight in the eyes, she said that. It felt like violation. [. . .]* (story 517) (Van Der Pijl et al., 2020, p. 13).

Although there are many more examples I could give from research on birth trauma, I acknowledge that they are difficult to read, especially if some of these examples are feeling like your own experience of birth trauma. Essentially, how you are treated and what you experience can all contribute to feelings of birth trauma, and all are valid. Let's move on to the impact of birth trauma.

Symptoms of Birth Trauma

Women can experience a range of symptoms following birth trauma. For some women, this can develop into a diagnosis of posttraumatic stress disorder (PTSD) or posttraumatic stress symptoms (PTSS) but many more can experience PTSD symptoms but be below the level of the diagnostic threshold (Ayers et al., 2015). The rate of women having diagnosed PTSD following childbirth is between 1% and 9% but is increased for women with risk factors, such as previous psychological diagnosis, previous experience of trauma and birth trauma (Anderson, 2017; Simpson et al., 2018).

Symptoms of PTSD are described in four groups: intrusions, avoidance, negative cognitions and mood, and hyperarousal. Ayers et al. (2018) developed a tool to measure the prevalence of PTSD following birth trauma based on the DSM-5 criteria. The DSM-5 is the current diagnostic and statistical manual used by mental health practitioners (APA, 2013). The City Birth Trauma Scale can be found through this link: https://www.frontiersin.org/articles/10.3389/fpsyt.2018.00409/full#supplementary-material

Throughout my qualitative research, I found quotes from women who experienced symptoms of birth trauma without having a formal mental health diagnosis. In the HBAC study, a woman described the impact on her sleep a month after her traumatic caesarean.

> *At about 4 weeks my primary midwife was talking to me about how I wasn't really sleeping, and she... helped me realise that it was me that was awake and not the baby, and that I was actually, like, replaying this surgery...that was what I was recalling, not the birth, but surgery, over and over in my mind and it made me sort of realise that I needed to speak to someone about it* (Mary) (Keedle et al., 2015, p. 5).

In the Journey meta-ethnography, a woman described the impact of her feelings after a traumatic caesarean.

> *At first, in the months after Harry was born, I lay awake in bed tearfully regaling Jo [husband] with my feelings of anger and regret and doubts. I'm mostly over the anger and regret now, but the doubts are still there* (Keedle et al., 2018b, p. 75)

Seeking Help

Personally, I feel that many women don't seek help after having a traumatic birth for many reasons. I think women who were belittled by healthcare providers during their birthing experience may feel disempowered and discouraged to seek help from the same or a different healthcare provider. Women are also often told "at least you have a healthy baby," which, other than stating the obvious, silences women. After all, how dare she complain about her traumatic birthing experience when her baby survived the process of extraction? The fact that she feels broken and abused is secondary to successfully producing a healthy baby, isn't it?

Becoming a mother is a transformative process, both physically, emotionally, and for some, spiritually. The process should be one that strengthens women to be able to nurture and care for their baby whilst acknowledging the amazing ability required during labour and birth. The impact of birth trauma is far reaching, not just for how the woman feels. It can impact bonding, breastfeeding, the ability to care for other children, relationships, and societal expectations. If women don't get help and remain silenced on their traumatic birthing experiences, then other women are not aware this can happen, or it becomes normalised. Get pregnant, listen to the horrific birthing experiences, be scared about the upcoming birth, accept everything the rushed healthcare provider says, have heaps of interventions, be disrespected, feel violated, have a horrific birthing experience, and the cycle continues. The cycle needs to be broken and there are ways this can occur.

An important step for women who have experienced birth trauma is to get professional help with a psychologist. There are many psychologists who have received extra training to work with women with birth trauma. In Australia, a great resource to go to is The Centre for Perinatal Psychology, where they have resources, a blog, and a list of psychologists across Australia https://www.centreforperinatalpsychology.com.au/

An international and U. S.-based support is the Birth & Trauma Support Center: https://birthandtraumasupportcenter.org/

Debriefing

The research on debriefing after a traumatic birth is divisive. A Cochrane review looking at randomised controlled trials on the effect of debriefing for the prevention of psychological trauma found no evidence to support routine debriefing, and that the studies found were small and too different to compare with each other (Bastos et al., 2015). To assume that debriefing alone will prevent psychological distress following an experience of birth trauma is like bolting the stable door once the horse has escaped. The experience of birth trauma happened. Debriefing can't rewind and stop the event from happening, but it might be able to help the woman understand what happened and why. This is understandably a delicate and important process that needs to be facilitated by skilled professionals and can be both structured or unstructured (Baxter, 2019).

A common practice in the hours or days after the birth is that a doctor from the obstetric medical team visits the woman and explains the reasons for the interventions required and then documents in the medical notes that the debrief has been completed. These visits rarely allow for the woman to ask questions or to voice how she feels, and the woman might not have had the opportunity to process any feelings, especially with the immediate requirements of looking after a newborn with little sleep.

Good debriefing can encourage women to reflect on their experience and gain clarification on the events that occurred. The woman should be able to explore what happened alongside others that witnessed it (the partner, for example), and the professional has the hospital notes to add information.

In research, women have found debriefing to be therapeutic, satisfying women's need to talk about the experience (Baxter et al., 2014), and validating (Inglis, 2002). Debriefing importantly gave women a voice and an opportunity to be listened to (Inglis, 2002) and improved clarity on reasons for caesarean (Dougan et al., 2019).

In my experience of debriefing as a private midwife, I have utilised a timeline, often starting the timeline in the last few days or weeks before labour started, and then adding the events the woman and partner remember. The notes help by adding times that interventions occurred. During the process, partners might remember things that happened that the woman doesn't, or the woman might mention how something made her feel that the partner wasn't aware of. Often, the addition of when interventions occurred started the realisation and knowledge about the cascade of intervention. The cascade of intervention describes the increased likelihood that the introduction of one medical or clinical intervention will lead to another intervention, each one negatively impacting the ability to have a vaginal birth.

I have found the debriefing process to be an important part of identifying the positive or negative impacts individuals and actions had on the traumatic experience. It isn't a process to portion blame but to gain understanding. By discussing the impact, the introduced intervention can have can give clarification to the woman and the partner, and hopefully lift the blame the woman often directs to herself.

Research has explored the timing of debriefing. Debriefing in the immediate postnatal period can feel overwhelming but may also be an opportunity to identify early concerns following a traumatic birth. An Australian study tested an early counselling intervention for women who reported a traumatic birthing experience (Gamble et al., 2005). The study was a randomized controlled trial, which meant that recruited women were randomly allocated to an intervention group or a control group. The intervention group was provided with two counselling sessions with trained midwives at 72 hours post-birth and at 4 to 6 weeks post-birth. The control group didn't receive counselling through the study. At 3 months post-birth, the women were scored for PTSD symptoms and depression. The intervention group had fewer PTSD symptoms, and low risk of depression and self-blame compared to the control group (Gamble et al., 2005).

The design of this study was recently replicated in Iran and again, the intervention group had less PTSD, depression, and anxiety compared to the control group (Asadzadeh et al., 2020). Both studies are relatively small, with 103 women in the Australian study and 90 women in the

Iranian study, which contributes to the lack of uptake of the model, but it certainly deserves further research and consideration.

An Irish study offered a debriefing service to women and found that on average, women contacted the service about a year after the traumatic birth experience, with some prompted as they were considering another pregnancy or were currently pregnant (Inglis, 2002). The anniversary of a traumatic birthing experience can be extremely difficult for women. Beck (2017) found that women described having to put on a mask during the celebrations of the child's birthday while feeling increased traumatic symptoms, such as flashbacks and increased anxiety.

Accessing Debriefing

There can be many challenges to access debriefing services, especially if you are no longer in the maternity service. First steps may include reaching out to the maternity unit and asking to speak to the midwifery manager. The manager may be able to meet or is aware of debriefing services in the area.

You may want to access your medical notes and have a debriefing with a midwife or doctor in the community. There are processes involved with accessing notes. Looking at your area health service website should help, as there is likely direction on how to access medical records. Occasionally, there is a fee, and you get limited information. I do suggest you go through these with a midwife or doctor to help with clarification and interpretation, and they may be able to help with context. Plus, debriefing is much more than just reading hospital notes, as has been discussed here.

Summary

Birth trauma is real and can have a detrimental impact on women, partners, and their families. Seeking help following an experience of birth trauma can be through formal therapy (counselling/psychology) and debriefing. Gaining knowledge on your previous caesarean experience can help you consider your choices for your next birth.

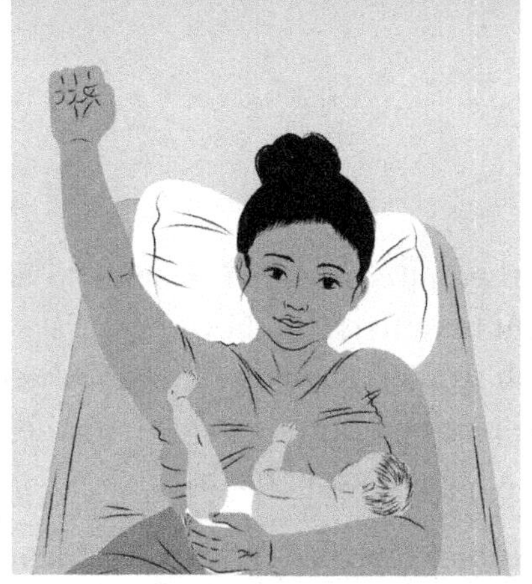

Chapter 3

YOUR BIRTH OPTIONS

Options

In this chapter I will explore the evidence around your different birth options and specific situations that may impact your decision making.

When you have had a previous caesarean, you have two options that will result in one of three outcomes. Planning an elective caesarean will result in an elective caesarean. Planning a VBAC can result in a VBAC, in an elective or emergency caesarean.

Table: Birth choices after caesarean

Planned birth choice	Actual mode of birth
Elective caesarean	Elective caesarean
Planned VBAC	VBAC
Planned VBAC	Emergency (unplanned) caesarean

Research shows us there are risks and benefits to each mode of birth. I think it is important to understand how these risks are presented and described in research studies; it comes down to whether they report on the outcomes of the planned groups (known as the intended mode of birth) and/or on the actual mode of births.

Some large earlier studies reported only on the intended mode of birth and reported the outcomes of these groups. This meant that the results of the intended elective caesarean group were compared to the intended VBAC group. However, in the intended VBAC group, there were women who had a repeat caesarean, often an emergency caesarean. This is not a fair comparison and sometimes the studies didn't publish the results of the actual mode of birth, making it difficult to know how the different outcomes of women who had a VBAC compared to having a caesarean. When you are deciding on what mode of birth after a previous caesarean you might want to know what those differences are; you understand planning a VBAC doesn't 100% guarantee having a VBAC.

One study that reported results of intended mode of birth was a South Australian study from 2012. Crowther (2012) found that women who intended to have a repeat elective caesarean had lower fetal and infant poor outcomes, and less severe post-birth bleeding rates compared to women who intended to have a VBAC. However, in the planned VBAC group, only 43% of women had a VBAC. The rest either had a repeat elective or emergency caesarean. I feel it doesn't really tell you the whole story. A couple of other large studies from the U. S. that also used this method of reporting outcomes based on intended mode of birth include Gilbert (2012) and Macones et al. (2005).

Recent studies have reported on the outcomes of the actual mode of birth, which means you can compare elective caesarean, emergency caesarean, and VBAC. Unfortunately, there outcomes are not consistent across studies, which I think shows the complexities of maternity care. A summary of the studies can be found in Table 1, where the differences that are statistically significant are reported. For a difference to be statistically significant means that the results are statistically different and not due to chance.

Table 1: Statistically significant differences between actual mode of birth

Study	Planned Elective CS	Planned VBAC had Emergency CS	Planned and had VBAC
Pont et al. (2018)	Requiring a blood transfusion		
	0.3%	1.2%	1.4%
Takeya et al. (2020)	Postpartum Haemorrhage		
	26%	20%	8%
Fitzpatrick et al. (2019)	Uterine rupture		
	0.04%	0.74%	0.04%
	Blood transfusion		
	0.5%	1.37%	1.05%
	Sepsis (Major infection)		
	0.17%	0.48%	0.18%
	Other infections		
	2.23%	4.29%	1.53%
	Exclusive breastfeeding at 6-8 weeks		
	24.94%	33.53%	33.57%
	Adverse outcome for baby		
	6.37%	10.33%	7.06%

As you can see from the above table, there are differences between modes of birth. These studies are based on large population data. Pont et al. (2018) reviewed 90,439 women's data from NSW, Australia, Takeya et al. (2020) reviewed 34,460 women's data from Japan, and Fitzpatrick et al. (2019) reviewed 74,043 women's data from Scotland. The rates of any of these outcomes occurring across the data is low, which is great. What can be seen is rates are highest in the emergency caesarean group for most of the outcomes. However, Takeya et al. (2020) found higher PPH rates and Fitzpatrick et al (2019) found lower exclusive breastfeeding rates at 6 to 8 weeks in the elective caesarean group.

These statistics only tell part of the story. They do not tell you how women felt after those birthing experiences, and I believe that is just as important. We will explore that further in other chapters.

Next, let us have a closer look at the risks of VBAC and then the risks of a repeat caesarean.

Risks of VBAC

Uterine Rupture

The most-feared risk of VBAC is uterine rupture. Fortunately, this is a rare event and not the reason most women have emergency caesareans when planning VBACs. When a woman has a lower segment transverse caesarean, an incision is made through the skin, abdominal muscles, and the three layers of the uterus. Following the caesarean, healing occurs in all levels, leaving a visible scar on the skin and a scar on the uterus.

A uterine rupture occurs when there is a separation through all three layers of the uterus. These layers are the endometrium (inner epithelial layer), myometrium (smooth muscle layer), and perimetrium (serosal outer surface) (Togioka & Tonismae, 2021). Uterine rupture can occur in women without a scar on their uterus and women with a scar due to any previous uterine surgery, including caesarean and myomectomy (removal of fibroids), and can occur during pregnancy or labour.

A uterine dehiscence, or partial rupture, is different from a complete uterine rupture due to being an incomplete separation that does not involve all three layers of the uterus.

> *Uterine dehiscence can produce a uterine window – a thinning of the uterine wall that may allow the foetus to be seen through the myometrium"* (Togioka & Tonismae, 2021, p. 1)

A dehiscence can be naturally occurring, incidental, and can be found during a repeat caesarean during labour. Previous obstetric care involved manual uterine examinations following a VBAC to check for ruptures, but thankfully, that invasive practice is no longer routine (Guiliano et al., 2014).

Uterine rupture is a rare occurrence. Internationally, rates of uterine rupture are consistently reported as less than 1% in the population of women birthing but let us take a closer look at those figures.

One of the largest uterine rupture studies to be reported is the International Network of Obstetric Survey Systems Study (INOSS) of uterine rupture, published in 2019. This multi-country population-based study reviewed data of 2,625,017 births across 9 European countries from 2004 to 2014 (Vandenberghe et al., 2019). From that large number of births, they found 864 women had complete uterine ruptures, which was a prevalence of 3.3 per 10,000 (0.03%) births. When they separated out women who had a previous caesarean from the population data of 2,625,017 births there were 743 uterine ruptures births, the rate of uterine rupture was 22 per 10,000 births, or 0.22%.

So, what happened to the women and babies because of uterine rupture?

In the cohort from Vandenberghe et al. (2019), there were 864 women who had a uterine rupture. Of those 864 women, 21% of women required more than 4 units of packed cells (4 bags of donated blood), 20% required an admission to intensive care, and 10% of women needed a hysterectomy. Two women out of 864 uterine ruptures died. While any death is terrible for the families of the women, the risk of death from uterine rupture is exceedingly low, 0.002%.

There were also good outcomes for most babies that were born during a uterine rupture. There was a 7.7% rate of babies who had asphyxia (deprivation of oxygen potentially causing harm). There were only 10% of babies that died during or as a result of uterine rupture.

To summarise, there will always be a small risk of having a uterine rupture when you have had a previous caesarean, but that risk is very small. If a woman does have a uterine rupture, it is unlikely she will die if she has timely access to urgent medical care and even then, 9 out of 10 babies born during a uterine rupture will survive.

Identifying a Uterine Rupture

A few studies have retrospectively looked at the onset and features of a uterine rupture. Guiliano et al. (2014) looked at 52 partial and complete uterine ruptures, and found several signs and symptoms were experienced, and these have also been found in the studies by Markou et al. (2017) and Chang (2020). These are listed in Table 2.

Table 2 – Signs of Uterine Rupture

Sign/Symptom	Guiliano et al. (2014) n=52	Chang et al. (2020) n=18	Markou et al. (2017) n=126
Fetal heart rate abnormality	46%	78%	47%
Abdominal pain	25%	28%	48%
Vaginal bleeding	23%	33%	30%
Loss of presentation	15%	-	-
Haematuria	4%	11%	-
Postpartum haemorrhage	14%	5%	-
Asymptomatic	33%	11%	-

These were not reported on in the study

The three most reported signs and symptoms of a uterine rupture during labour include a fetal heart rate abnormality, abdominal pain (different or on top of contraction pain), and abnormal vaginal bleeding. Fetal heart rate abnormalities (FHR) often presented as the onset of persistent bradycardia (continuous low heart rate) (Guiliano et al., 2014) and is the reasoning given for including cardiotocography (CTG) monitoring in VBAC policies and guidelines.

Whether intermittent monitoring using a doppler can pick up the same FHR abnormalities is an area not researched. However, a large Cochrane systematic review of studies comparing continuous CTG monitoring to intermittent monitoring found no difference in the numbers of babies who died but continuous CTG monitoring did increase intervention and caesarean rates (Alfirevic et al., 2017).

Following a Uterine Rupture

A few studies have explored the impact of a previous uterine rupture on future birthing options. A small study from the U.S. looked at the outcomes of 20 women who had a prior uterine rupture, and 40 women who had a prior uterine dehiscence. All women had a repeat elective caesarean with most being between 36 to 39 weeks gestation with 6.7% of women having a uterine dehiscence identified during their repeat elective caesarean (Fox et al., 2014).

The same cohort of women alongside other reported incidences of uterine rupture or dehiscence were examined 5 years later. Many of the women went on to have more than one subsequent pregnancies, and it was found that 12% of all the pregnancies had an observed uterine dehiscence at the time of the repeat elective caesarean, with one case of a repeat uterine rupture (Fox, 2020).

The authors surmised that women with a previous uterine rupture or dehiscence should have a repeat elective caesarean before the onset of spontaneous labour, yet there are no published studies that compare the outcomes of women with a previous complete or partial uterine rupture who have a vaginal birth compared to having a caesarean.

The standard advice given to women following a uterine rupture is to have an elective caesarean at 37 to 38 weeks of their next pregnancy. There is little research on women's experiences of planning a VBAC after a rupture (VBAR) but there are women who wish to have this experience. One woman who experienced a VBAR is Kari Lammer from Iowa in the USA. Her full story is available in Chapter 10.

Kari experienced a uterine rupture during her VBAC birth, which was diagnosed on Day 3 while she was rooming in with her baby in NICU. Although it was scary and traumatic, Kari describes her feelings about this experience and her wishes for subsequent pregnancies below.

For me, it was an ideal birth, minus the rupture. Despite the rupture, I had an amazing birth high. As to why the first c-section was more traumatic than the vaginal birth with a rupture, I don't know. I wonder if it has to do with the lack of control or a feeling of being taken advantage of (my fault for not being educated going into our first birth) from that c-section? Maybe it's simply the memory of being alone, the all-white-sterile room, not being able to see my baby. I'm just not sure.

We were undecided on a third going into our second birth, but with the rupture, there was even more to question if we were to have another. A hysterectomy was not needed; I was told I could have more children but would need to be delivered between 37 to 38 weeks via scheduled c-section.

Regardless, I knew if we had a third, I wanted another VBAC/VBAR. I joined the Special Scars Facebook group and learned of many people who go on to have vaginal births after doctors told them it wasn't possible based on their birth history. When I shared my story, I learned of a clinic that supported VBARs. I learned a ton more than that, but knowing it was possible gave me hope.

I did all sorts of things to prepare for a third baby, should we make that decision. I started seeing a therapist who specializes in birthing trauma. I started collagen and vitamin C supplements to strengthen my uterus. I read every piece of literature or study on pregnancy after rupture and/or ruptures in general. I joined a Facebook group that is for people who are interested in a vaginal birth post-rupture. It's not just me who wants this!"

Risks of Elective/Emergency Caesarean

A caesarean is major abdominal surgery. Having a caesarean has the risk of both short-term and long-term complications. Earlier in the chapter, we explored the complications of post-birth bleeding and infections following a caesarean. In this section, we will explore long-term complications and the potential impact of caesareans on infants and children.

Long-Term Complications

Abnormalities of Placentation

The wall of the uterus consists of three layers. The placenta invades and attaches to the endometrium layer of the uterus but in some pregnancies, there can be an abnormal attachment of the placenta to the uterine wall, and this is called placenta-accreta spectrum. Placenta accreta occurs when the placenta implants in the deeper myometrium muscle layer of the uterus. The severity of the accreta depends on the depth of this attachment (Clark, 2011; Pairman et al., 2019).

Rates of placenta accreta have increased in conjunction with rising caesarean rates and increase for women with multiple pregnancies (Clark, 2011). Due to the deeper implantation of the placenta, women are at higher risks of significant bleeding after placenta separation and the rates of needing a blood transfusion or requiring a hysterectomy are higher with placenta accreta.

The more caesareans the woman has, the greater her chance of experiencing placenta accreta in a subsequent pregnancy. The risk of experiencing placenta accreta following one caesarean is 3%, 11% following the second, 40% for the third, 60% for the fourth, and for five or more caesareans the risk raises to 67% (Sandall et al., 2018).

Adhesions

> *Abdominal/pelvic adhesions are fibrous, band-like structures that form between abdominal organs or between the peritoneum and abdominal wall when trauma induces inflammation and disrupts normal tissue* (Lyell, 2011, p. S11).

Women can develop adhesions following a caesarean and these adhesions can result in chronic scar or abdominal pain, pain with bowel movements, and pain with sexual activity (Wasserman et al., 2018). Pelvic adhesions increase the risk for secondary infertility and ectopic pregnancy. Subsequent caesareans for women with adhesions can result in more surgical complications and higher rates of infection (Saban et al., 2019).

If you think you might be experiencing difficulties with chronic abdominal/pelvic pain following a caesarean, you should discuss this with your General Practitioner or healthcare provider. There are some treatments available, such as soft-tissue mobilisation, physical therapy, and medication (Wasserman et al., 2018).

The Impact of Caesarean on Infants/Children

There is limited research on the impact of interventions and type of birth on infant and children's wellbeing. A U.S. study looked at the outcomes for 22,690 children born by VBAC or caesarean in relation to rates of otitis media (ear infections), respiratory infections, and food allergies (Kikuchi et al., 2020). Kikuchi et al. (2020) found that 2-year-old children born by caesarean had a significantly higher risk of developing otitis media and respiratory infections, but there was no difference in food allergies. However, in this study there was no available data on social and behavioural factors such as smoking and breastfeeding (Kikuchi et al. 2020).

A small study from the Czech Republic conducted cognitive tests on 5-year-old children who were born either by caesarean or vaginal birth (Blazkova et al., 2020). Blazkova et al. (2020) found children born vaginally had higher cognitive development performance than children born via caesarean, which was further pronounced in boys versus girls. There was no change in the results when length of breastfeeding was included. Maternal mental health was not reported on in this study. This study is small, however; only 169 children were included in the 5-year follow up tests.

To summarise, having a caesarean is having major abdominal surgery and may have short- and long-term physical complications. These complications can impact women's quality of life, such as pain from adhesions, and impact the next pregnancy and birthing experience. However, not all women will experience physical complications.

VBAC Rates

After looking at the risks of planning a VBAC compared to planning an elective caesarean it might be surprising to learn that most women with a previous caesarean have repeat caesareans for their subsequent births. In both the U. S. and Australia, 86% of women have a repeat caesarean (AIHW, 2020; Martin et al., 2018). That makes roughly 1 in 8 women who have a previous caesarean having a VBAC for their next birth. These national statistics do not indicate how many women planned a VBAC and had a repeat caesarean, only the outcome of the birth.

National guidelines and policies have impacted VBAC rates. In 1999 The American College of Obstetricians and Gynecologists (ACOG) published guidelines that dramatically decreased VBAC rates. The guidelines stated that VBAC should only be attempted in institutions that had immediate access to emergency care. Smaller and rural hospitals across the USA who didn't have on-site anaesthetists and operating theatre staff ceased supporting women planning a VBAC and by 2004 the VBAC rate dropped to 9.2% (Roberts et al., 2007). Professional organisations in other countries followed the new ACOG guidelines, including Australia.

In a more positive move, the recent ACOG guidelines released in 2017 state that most women with a previous low-transverse incision should have the right to plan a VBAC, with consideration of coinciding potentially complicating factors. These guidelines will be explored further in this book. In the UK the recent National Institute for Health and Care Excellence (NICE) guidelines (2019) supported access to water immersion and to not routinely offer intravenous cannulation. Unfortunately, there is currently a lack of progressive guidelines around VBAC to emerge from Australia.

VBAC rates vary internationally with some European countries, such as Finland having VBAC rates as high as 55% and as low as Cyprus, with 4.7% (Euro-Peristat Project, 2018). In China, where the universal two-child policy was introduced in 2016 and maternal requested caesarean rates are high (Yu et al., 2017), a study gave a VBAC rate of 9.6% (Mu et al., 2018).

I feel there is a lot to learn from the vast variety in VBAC rates internationally. Around the world, women can get pregnant and give birth vaginally. The difference is the system that they birth in. There are many global health inequalities and differences in maternity care between low- and high-resource countries (SoWMy, 2021) yet the differences in VBAC rates in high-resource countries suggest the influence of the maternity care system, guiding policies, the model of care, and the healthcare professional as more influential than the differences between women.

This is where women can make important choices. Depending on your circumstances, you can choose the model of care and/or healthcare professional that will best support *you* to plan the best birth for you. We will explore this further in Chapter 6.

Length of Time Between Caesarean and the Next Birth

The length of time between the previous caesarean and the next birth is known as the interdelivery interval, and the time between the previous caesarean and conception of the next pregnancy is known as the interpregnancy interval. Research explores the outcomes for women planning a VBAC with short- and long-time intervals between the births in relation to uterine rupture risk.

Original research by Stamilio (2007) in the USA evaluated the interpregnancy interval outcomes at less than 6 months, from 6 months to 12 months, and from 12 months to 18 months in 13,331 women. For women with less than 6 months, the uterine rupture risk was 2.7% and the need blood transfusion rate was 2.4% compared with women of 6 or more months who had a uterine rupture risk of 0.9% and blood transfusion rate of 0.7% (Stamilio, 2007). The VBAC rate was 77% and this was consistent across the different interpregnancy time frames (Stamilio, 2007).

A similar study of 36,653 women from the Netherlands found no increased uterine rupture rate across interpregnancy intervals, with rates ranging from 0.16-0.26% (Rietveld et al., 2017). VBAC rates were

72% for women with intervals less than 24 months and 67% for longer intervals (Rietveld et al., 2017).

Women are often discouraged from planning a VBAC when they have interpregnancy intervals of less than 12 to 18 months, yet the research doesn't show dramatic changes in uterine rupture rates for shorter interpregnancy intervals. The shortest interval investigated, which was less than 6 months between the caesarean and conception, increased the rupture rate to 2.7% in the U. S. study (Stamilio, 2007) and remained less than 1% in the study from the Netherlands (Rietveld et al., 2017). If we take the conservative number of 2.7%, that means, even in the worst case scenario, there is a 97.3% chance of not having a uterine rupture. Remember, once the interpregnancy interval passes 6 months those rates decrease significantly. It doesn't mean you are absolutely going to have a rupture, and a healthcare professional can't state that or use coercion on you due to those risks.

Personally, I was in the interpregnancy interval of less-than-6-months group, and I was confident in focusing on the 97.3% chance of not having a uterine rupture. At 13 months after my caesarean, I had a VBAC without a uterine rupture.

You will need to come to your own decisions about what risk level you are comfortable with and then plan for the best birth for *you*.

VBAC Calculators

I just want to add my thoughts about VBAC prediction tools and the VBAC calculator. It is fair to say I am not a fan and that is because they don't include some of the biggest influencers on VBAC rates.

The VBAC calculator was designed by Grobman et al. (2007) to assist clinicians in predicting what types of women were likely to have a VBAC. From reviewing the data of 7,660 women who had a previous caesarean and had a subsequent birth, the researcher found six variables that impacted VBAC rates. These were age, BMI, ethnicity, vaginal birth since caesarean, any history of vaginal birth, and whether the reason for the caesarean is deemed as potentially recurrent (Grobman et al., 2007).

This VBAC calculator has been validated, reproduced, adapted, and tested in a variety of different languages and countries, and is available as an app for clinicians and women to use (Fagerberg et al., 2015; Lakra et al., 2020; Mooney et al., 2019).

So, if it has been so well researched and used in multiple different countries, why am I not a fan? It is due to the addition of social constructs of race and ethnicity, and the omission of healthcare providers attitudes and maternity system differences that make the VBAC calculator flawed. This has been described by Thornton (2018):

> *This calculator has significant limitations that are easily overlooked by women and providers alike. The calculator has much greater positive than negative predictive power, and it cannot predict unsuccessful TOLAC or uterine rupture. Furthermore, the calculator cannot predict rare catastrophes, such as unplanned hysterectomy, permanent injury, or death. Predictions are heavily influenced by race and ethnicity, which are social and not biological constructs. Relevant variables, such as provider attitudes and institutional differences, are not accounted for. Providers should be mindful and transparent about calculator limitations when counselling women, particularly Latina and African American women. It may be appropriate to use the calculator to inform but not restrict women's options* (Thornton, 2018, p. 115).

The concerns of Thornton and other researchers (Vyas et al., 2019) were considered by the original calculator team and a newer updated version was released that removed race and ethnicity, and included chronic hypertension (Grobman et al., 2021). Out of interest, I did the new calculator based on my information when I did plan a VBAC, and my predicted chance was 51.6%, but since I had a short interpregnancy interval, I was strongly advised against having a VBAC. I did it anyway.

An obstetrician researcher who has conducted his PhD on the use of the VBAC calculator in California is quoted in a news article on the calculator.

Nicholas Rubashkin, a clinical professor of obstetrics, gynecology, and reproductive sciences at UCSF, also noted that the calculator is still a black box. "While this new calculator doesn't include race/ethnicity, the authors didn't tell us about the distribution of racial/ethnic groups across the score ranges," he said in an email. And even a de-racialized tool can reinforce care discrepancies if it is not used carefully. While the calculator was never intended to be a screening tool, Rubashkin's research indicates some physicians use a VBAC calculator result of 60% to 70% as a cut-off, refusing to offer the option to patients who score lower.

'There's still more work that needs to be done to undo the harms of having this tool out in the world since 2007,' said Rubashkin." (Palmer, 2021).

Another issue with the VBAC calculator is that is removes the influence of the healthcare provider, model of care, and maternity system from the calculation. There is plenty of research that identifies the benefits of midwifery models of care (Sandall et al., 2016), which will be explored further in Chapter 6, and there are smaller studies available that show the positive impact of midwifery models of care on VBAC rates (Rosenstein et al., 2015; Zhang & Liu, 2016). Birth location also impacts VBAC rates with out-of-hospital births having higher VBAC rates than hospital births (Beckmann et al., 2014; Cheyney et al., 2014).

If you are in an appointment with a healthcare provider who uses the VBAC calculator and gives you a 60% VBAC chance, but they personally don't believe in or support VBAC, and use interventions and coercion to dissuade you from VBAC, then your 60% VBAC rate is more like 1% if you stay with that provider. Therefore, choosing your team is vital and we will explore this in Chapter 6.

Summary

This chapter has explored the current research and literature on birth options after caesarean, along with myth busting common restrictions given to women who wish to plan a VBAC.

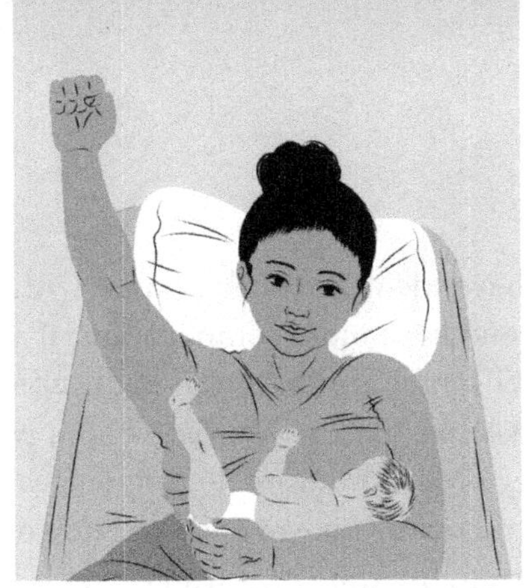

Chapter 4

CAN I HAVE A VBAC IF...?

In this chapter I will explore the different situations you may be experiencing that may lead you to ask the question, "Can I have a VBAC if...?"

The topics I will explore are larger women (higher BMI), induction of labour, multiple pregnancy (twins, etc.), breech presentation, more than one previous caesarean, special scars, and place of birth. I will weave in women's stories either from my research studies or shared with me, alongside the current research on the topic.

"I Have a Higher BMI"

Women who have a higher BMI (≥30kg/m^2) frequently experience stigma and weight bias from healthcare professionals (Mulherin et al., 2013). A study from the USA that interviewed women who experienced weight stigma found the women experienced judgement, stereotyping, bullying, and coercion when accessing maternity care (Dejoy et al., 2016).

Once you add planning a VBAC on top of weight stigma, you can only imagine the pressure and disrespectful care that women could receive but is there a valid reason why women with a higher BMI shouldn't plan a VBAC?

Research studies have identified that women with a higher BMI have lower VBAC rates and have more complications if an emergency caesarean is required (Wilson et al., 2020; Yao et al., 2019). However, a study from the USA that looked at the outcome of 614 women found that in women with higher BMI there were no differences in VBAC rates (Mei et al., 2019). The American College of Obstetricians and Gynecologists (ACOG) guidelines of 2017 state that women with a BMI of 30 or more can plan a VBAC, but their care should be individualised (ACOG, 2017).

As women with higher BMI's have higher prevalence of surgical complications, such as wound infections and venous clots, it is understandable why planning a VBAC would be a safer choice. This needs to be balanced with understanding the risks associated with needing a repeat emergency caesarean. Understanding your options, choosing your team, and being aware how to plan for the best birth for you is essential.

Some women find that their BMI isn't directly referred to by healthcare professionals and others find it is mentioned in the first appointment. Hannah Archer from Victoria in Australia found it was mentioned in her first phone appointment with a midwife. Hannah's full story can be found in Chapter 10.

> *My first appointment was a phone appointment with a midwife who recommended I get an early GDM [gestational diabetes] test, as I had a high BMI of close to 40. They also said they would bring me up in a meeting. There's a technical term for it but I can't remember what the meeting is called. It was decided that I should take blood thinners, as my higher BMI could supposedly mean my placenta and cord might not function correctly and the baby might end up with restricted growth. In the same breath, I was also told that I would need to have growth scans at 28, 32, and 36 weeks, due to my BMI and fear of large baby. After consideration, I decided against the blood thinners.*

"I Need to Be Induced"

Being induced refers to having labour started before the body has started labour. There are a variety of methods to start labour, and these can include medication and manual interventions. Initial methods may include the use of vaginal pessaries, gel, or tape that have synthetic hormones, such as prostaglandin, and/or having a "stretch and sweep" vaginal examination, where a midwife or doctor locates the cervix with their fingers and attempts to gently widen the cervix and perform a sweeping action with the fingers to agitate the amniotic membranes. Sometimes, a catheter with a balloon is inserted into the vagina, the balloon is filled with sterile water, and this sits in the cervix, helping it to open.

Many women experience artificial rupture of membranes (ARM) to induce labour. This is where a doctor or midwife performs a vaginal examination and uses an instrument with a small hook on the end to break the waters.

The synthetic version of the labour hormone oxytocin, known as Syntocinon or Pitocin, is also used to induce labour and to augment labour. Augmentation is used when labour has started naturally but there are concerns about the progress or strength of contractions. Synthetic oxytocin is delivered via an intravenous (IV) cannula and IV machine (pump) and started on a low dose and increased slowly until the contractions are strong and regular, around 3-4 contractions every 10 minutes. Increasing synthetic oxytocin too quickly can result in uterine hyperstimulation, where the uterus is contracting too much, and this can be a risk to the woman and the baby.

There are a variety of views around induction and VBAC. Some hospitals and healthcare providers won't offer induction to women planning a VBAC or they will only use certain induction methods and not others. This is due to the impact induction of labour can have on uterine rupture rates and on VBAC rates.

Early research into induction and VBAC found slightly higher uterine rupture rates when prostaglandin gel alone or a combination of prostaglandin gel and synthetic oxytocin was used (Buhimschi et al., 2005; Dekker, 2010; Stock et al., 2013), which led to prostaglandin gel not being recommended for women planning a VBAC.

Recent research has explored the use of balloon catheters for induction in women planning a VBAC. A small study of 1,920 women from France compared the VBAC rates of women who had a balloon catheter and synthetic oxytocin to women who had synthetic oxytocin alone (Secchi et al., 2021). They found 61% of women in the balloon group had a VBAC compared to 48% of women in the synthetic oxytocin-alone group. There were four uterine ruptures in the balloon group and eight in the oxytocin alone group (Secchi et al., 2021). A small study of 208 women in the UK comparing the use of the balloon catheter to the use of prostaglandin gel found no significant differences between the two groups and VBAC rates of 53% in the balloon group and 67% in the prostaglandin group, and most women in both groups also had synthetic oxytocin (Bullough et al., 2021).

The American College of Obstetricians and Gynecologists (ACOG) note that there is a variety of research on the use of induction of labour and VBAC. They recommend the use of balloon catheters but identify it is difficult to give a definitive recommendation on the use of prostaglandin. Regarding the use of synthetic oxytocin, they conclude that:

> *... given that the results of these studies vary and that the absolute magnitude of the risk reported in these studies is small, oxytocin augmentation may be used in women [planning a VBAC]* (ACOG, 2017, p. e222).

The decision to have an induction of labour when planning a VBAC can be a complicated one. The alternative to induction is waiting for labour to start spontaneously (naturally) or having a repeat elective caesarean. As discussed in the previous chapter, there are risks to both options and you will need to explore which option feels right for you. Discuss this with your team and think about it in your birth plan (we will look at birth plans in the next chapter).

"I Have Gestational Diabetes Mellitus (GDM)"

There are few studies that have explored women's experiences of planning a VBAC and having gestational diabetes together. A small study from Israel found the women with GDM with a previous caesarean were generally a little older and had a higher pre-pregnancy BMI compared to the women who didn't have GDM (Ganer Herman et al., 2017). Ganer Herman et al. (2017) also found more women with GDM had a repeat caesarean compared to women without GDM and women with a previous VBAC had higher VBAC rates in both groups.

As GDM rates increase alongside caesarean rates, we can expect many women to be considering their birth after caesarean options while having GDM. Women with GDM are often given a lot of unnecessary pressure regarding inductions and interventions, which make planning a VBAC challenging. It can be done though, and Chapter 10 has 14 stories from women who had a VBAC while also having GDM.

Hannah experienced repeat GDM while planning a VBAC and she initially felt pressure by the obstetric doctor at her local, smaller, hospital to transfer to the larger hospital due to GDM and her BMI.

> *At my first meeting with one of the obstetricians (small country hospital so no option for continued care; you just get who you get), she said "you've got GDM. You best go to the metropolitan hospital 30 mins away, cause you'll most likely end up on insulin and end up there anyway." I said "no thanks, I would like to see how I go." In the same conversation, she weighed me and checked my BMI, and said "you're going to go over on your BMI, so you should probably just go to the metropolitan hospital, because you're going to put on weight and end up there anyway." I sort of just sat there and waited for her to talk. She told me to come back in 4 weeks, and we'll re-evaluate. Four weeks later, and I had lost half a kilo. I wished so bad that the obstetrician would be on that day, but she wasn't.*

"My Baby is Breech"

Many women have experienced a caesarean for a breech presentation, which was certainly my experience. Thankfully, the tide is slowly turning with the reintroduction of vaginal breech birth in some hospitals, which will in turn, mean more women who have had a previous caesarean will be exploring their birthing options if they have a breech presentation in their next pregnancy.

During pregnancy, women who have a breech presentation are often offered an external cephalic version (ECV), which is a manual rotation of the baby from bottom down to head down. In the past, there has been hesitancy from obstetric doctors in offering ECV to women who have had a previous caesarean. However, recent ACOG guidelines recognise that women with a previous caesarean are not contraindicated to be offered an ECV and that success rates in rotating from breech to head down are similar when compared with women without a previous caesarean (ACOG, 2017).

It can be difficult to find supportive healthcare providers who will conduct an ECV for women with a previous caesarean. Siobhan had three breech pregnancies. Her full story is available in Chapter 10. In her first pregnancy, she had a painful and unsuccessful ECV and had a caesarean for breech presentation. During her second pregnancy, she was planning a VBAC and when her baby turned to breech presentation, she used the internet to find a supportive doctor who would do an ECV.

> *The time was approaching for when I could attempt an ECV. I kept seeing stories of this amazing doctor (practically the breech baby whisperer) turning all these babies and supporting breech birth for those he could not turn. He was in Sydney, and I was on the Gold Coast. It would be mad for me to try and go see him, right?*
>
> *Well, I made a phone call to the Royal Hospital for Women and spoke with Dr Bisits, and he agreed to see me. So, 37 weeks pregnant with my toddler in tow, we flew to Sydney to see him for an ECV. The procedure took barely minutes and was no more than slightly uncomfortable. It was a completely opposite experience to the attempt with my son. He did it! She turned! I finally had a baby head down. Four weeks later, at 40w + 8d, I had my empowering VBAC.*

To date, there are few studies that have explored the outcome for women with a breech presentation planning a VBAC. A small study from Germany, which included 37 women with a previous caesarean, found no difference in outcomes for the women or babies and that the VBAC rate was also similar, concluding that vaginal breech birth was suitable for women with a previous caesarean (Paul et al., 2020). This study was small and further studies are required to understand the outcomes for women and babies, but it is a reassuring start.

In Chapter 10, Hayley shares her experience of having a breech VBAC in Sydney, Australia. I love this section where she describes the moment her baby is born, legs first.

> *I was so shocked later to learn that my baby was hanging out of me by his head at that point. With the next contraction, I made the wailing noise. Sam told me to concentrate on pushing, not yelling, so I closed my mouth and pushed where I assumed the pressure should be, and in the next moment, my giant 4.2 kg baby was splattered on my chest, angry crying, covered in meconium all over his body and his head was bright red with my blood. I was so shocked, as even though I knew that he must be nearly out, because I couldn't feel any sensations, I just wasn't ready to have a baby on me. Everyone gasped because he was so big, but he just looked normal to me.*

"I Am Pregnant with Twins"

To date, there is limited research available for the outcomes for women planning a VBAC when pregnant with twins. A systematic review that included 10 studies found similar VBAC rates in women pregnant with twins when compared to women pregnant with one baby and that there were significantly lower infections rates in the VBAC group compared to the repeat caesarean group (Shinar et al., 2019).

Although this review found a higher perinatal mortality rate in the VBAC group, the authors suggested this could be influenced by the higher premature births that can occur with twin pregnancies (Shinar et al., 2019). This trend hasn't been found in other published studies, such as the study by Varner et al. (2007), which found women pregnant with multiples had high VBAC rates and low complications rates. The ACOG (2017) guidelines are supportive of women pregnant with twins to plan a VBAC.

"I've Had More than One Caesarean"

The research on women who have had two or more caesareans is largely positive. Modzelewski et al. (2019) explored the experiences of women who had two previous caesareans in a small study from Poland. Only 8% (n=35) of women planned a VBAC after two caesareans (VBA2C) and 22 of the women had a VBA2C (63%). For women who had a VBAC, there were lower maternal and perinatal morbidity outcomes (Modzelewski et al., 2019). To put this study into perspective, they looked at 47,011 women and only 35 women planned a VBA2C. This doesn't surprise me that much; it is difficult for women to get support for a VBAC after two or more caesareans, even when the research is favourable.

A systematic review of 17 studies included 5,666 women planning a VBAC after multiple caesareans found an average VBAC rate of 71%, a uterine rupture rate of 1.36%, and similar neonatal and maternal outcomes between VBA2C and repeat caesarean (Tahseen & Griffiths, 2010). AGOC (2017) guidelines state that it is reasonable for women with two previous caesareans to plan a VBAC.

Cahill et al. (2010) explored the outcomes for women who planned a VBAC after three or more caesareans. From 860 women, the study found VBAC rates of 80%, no uterine ruptures, and no difference in maternal morbidity outcomes.

Planning a VBAC after two or more caesareans takes a large amount of courage and determination, as women can experience copious amounts of negativity and limitations from healthcare providers. Women can also feel double the amount of doubt in the ability of their body to birth.

Erin explains below her feelings about her body after her two caesareans and why and how she planned for her homebirth after them (HBA2C). Her full story is in Chapter 10.

> *My first two daughters were both born by caesarean. The first was a classic failure to progress, or failure to wait. I planned a homebirth with my second, but after four days of labour, my waters broke with thick meconium. I transferred to hospital, labour stalled, and after several hours, the baby started to show signs of distress. They were both big babies. They both went from more favourable to less favourable positions during labour or shortly before. Neither of them ever engaged in my pelvis. I thought my body was truly a lemon. I could blame the hospital for my first surgery, but after my second surgery,*

when I had planned a homebirth and completely trusted the process, I felt the buck stopped with me. And I had failed.

I wanted a third child, but I was scared to conceive again. I was scared that I wanted another chance to birth naturally, instead of another baby. I was scared of going through the whole emotional journey again, only to fail again. Samara got tired of waiting for me to work it out; her conception was a happy surprise for us! I planned a homebirth—of course I did. I don't have it in me to choose caesarean. I believe the way we are born matters. Deep in my soul, somewhere, I knew what birth was supposed to be like. I had to try again, though for the first time, I had no belief in my body. I was lucky enough to be able to surround myself with three wonderful women—two midwives and a doula—who did all the believing for me." Erin Quinn

"I Have a Special Scar"

A special scar includes women who had a variety of caesarean scars that were not lower uterine transverse scar (LSCS). These include:

» J incisions

» Inverted T

» Classical scar

» Low vertical

» Upright T

» Lower uterine extended

» Previous uterine rupture

These different types of incisions may be due to a variety of reasons and emergencies, such as prematurity, transverse position, adhesions, resources, and situation. Women with a special scar are usually advised to have a repeat caesarean at 37 to 38 weeks to prevent uterine rupture due to increased pressure and stretching of the uterus. However, women with a special scar often wish to have a VBAC and their wishes and decisions should be respected.

There is some research available on the outcomes of women with a special scar, although the studies are not current. A study from the USA compared the operative outcomes of 122 women with a classical scar to 7,814 women with an LSCS and found 12% of women with a classical scar had a repeat classical incision (Bakhshi et al., 2010). All women planned a repeat caesarean; there were no women who planned a VBAC. Women with a classical scar had longer operative time and hospital stay, higher intensive care unit admission, and more frequent uterine dehiscence (Bakhshi et al., 2010). An earlier study comparing 157 women with a classical scar to women with a LSCS had similar findings with a *dehiscence* rate of 9% (Chauhan et al., 2002). Remember that a dehiscence isn't a full uterine rupture and in all the research available of women who had repeat caesareans, there isn't recent research available to compare women with classical caesarean scar planning a VBAC.

ACOG (2017) guidelines suggest that for women with a previous low vertical scar, the evidence doesn't suggest increased rupture or morbidity risk, and that women may choose to plan a VBAC. Women with a previous classical or T incision, or previous uterine rupture are not encouraged to plan a VBAC according to the ACOG (2017) guidelines, yet there is limited data on the outcomes for women who have different types of scars, including inverted T scars. A couple of studies had women in their cohort that had inverted T scars and had a VBAC, but the numbers are too small to see any significant outcomes or comparisons (Kwee et al., 2007; Patterson et al., 2002).

Naomi from New Zealand had a caesarean for her first baby due to breech presentation and the baby not descending while being supported for a breech vaginal birth. She describes what she was told by the obstetrician. Her full story is in Chapter 10.

> *The next morning, the obstetrician came to see me and explained that it was a difficult surgery. The baby's head was entrapped under my ribs and was unable to be extracted, even with the extension of the transverse incision. He then made an incision 8 cm vertically to form an inverted T. It was still difficult to birth the baby, so forceps were needed. The baby came out and needed to be resuscitated but was able to come and meet me within 10 minutes. I cried when I heard about the*

complications of my surgery, as I knew that the recommendation was for all future births to be elective caesareans.

The healing, both mentally and physically, was hard, but I made an effort to not push myself physically and allow myself to feel all the raw emotions and grieve my lost homebirth that I had envisioned.

Caroline from the UK had a classical caesarean scar due to prematurity and a transverse position. Caroline wanted a VBAC for her next birth and experienced negativity when she saw an obstetric doctor.

I went to see the consultant who delivered Sophie and was there when I was on the antenatal ward. He told me that no obstetrician would let me deliver naturally again. I would have to have a planned c-section. I thought "on your bike, mate."

For her next pregnancy, she hired independent midwives and they informed her about the special scar's organisation.

They gave me information about the special scars Facebook group, and I got lots of information and support from them. I was able to chat to lots of other mums who had done what I was planning to do and totally understood all the scare tactics the medics were giving me. About how I could die, and I was being reckless. They gave me the percentages about the risk of uterine rupture up to 10% depending on what research you read. Well, turn that on its head and it's a 90% chance of it not happening.

You can read Hannah's whole story in Chapter 10.

Special Scars – Special Hope, a non-profit, volunteer-led organisation, supporting individuals on their special scar journeys through private social media support pages, is an invaluable resource for women with a special scar. More information can be found via their website: https://specialscars.org/

"I Choose to Birth at Home or in a Birth Centre"

My first research project was my master's honours, where I did a qualitative study into women's experiences of planning a VBAC at home (HBAC) in Australia. I had a keen interest in this topic, as I had planned a VBAC at home but transferred to hospital, as my team was unavailable. I was also a private midwife offering homebirth.

I interviewed 12 women who had all had a HBAC and the overarching theme was, "It [a caesarean] will never happen again." The women shared with me their often-traumatic previous caesareans and how they came to deciding on a HBAC. Their stories were full of trying to negotiate with hospitals about avoiding certain interventions but being told to agree to their policies or go away. This often led them to finding a privately practicing midwife, who would change the dialogue from "no, you can't" to "yes, you can." The women found healing and joy in their HBAC and the theme, "I felt like Superwoman," described the reactions I got from women when I asked them, "how did you feel after your VBAC at home?"

Birthing at home or at a birth centre has many benefits, including higher VBAC rates compared to hospital VBAC rates (Bayrampour et al., 2021; Beckmann et al., 2014; Latendresse, 2005). However, a population-based study from the USA found a higher intrapartum fetal death rate in women planning a HBAC (0.29%) compared to women without a previous caesarean birthing at home (0.06%), although the three deaths were not related to uterine rupture (Cheyney et al., 2014). A Canadian study found a HBAC rate of 86% compared to a VBAC in hospital rate of 70%, and that adverse outcomes were rare in both groups and not different between home and hospital (Bayrampour et al., 2021).

Adverse outcomes can occur during labour and birth, regardless of location, and when they occur, they need early recognition, assessment, and treatment. Midwives are trained to recognise and treat many adverse outcomes and can transfer the woman to hospital when required. The woman and their midwife need to have open and honest conversations about the potential for transfer based on their location and services available.

Summary

This chapter has explored the different scenarios that may have led to you asking, "Can I have a VBAC if...?" Remember, it should be only *you* who can answer that question for *you*, but hopefully, this chapter has increased your knowledge, which can assist you in making an informed decision.

I will now move on to the findings from my PhD, which were the four factors that impacted how a woman felt after her birthing experience following a previous caesarean. These factors are having control, having confidence, having a relationship, and having an active labour.

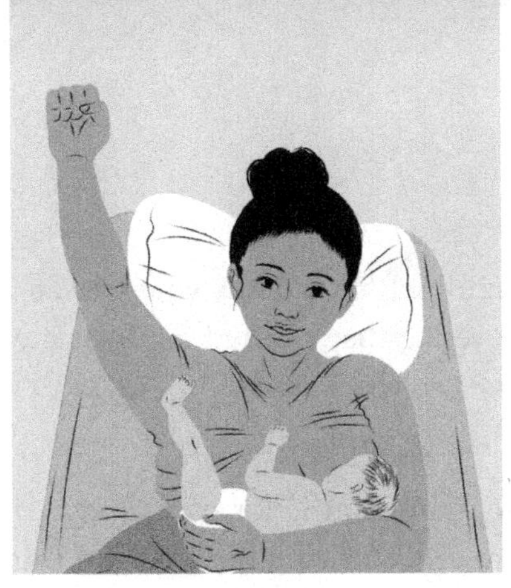

Chapter 5

HAVING CONTROL

Introduction

The first factor that contributes to whether a woman feels resolved or disappointed following a planned VBAC is "having control." The definition for "having control" is when a woman felt her wishes and choices were respected, and that she felt in control of her pregnancy and birthing decisions and outcomes. Feeling "out of control" contributes to birth trauma, as was discussed in Chapter 2.

It is important to put some context into why women feel out of control in the maternity care system and the reasons relate to the systemic prejudices and patriarchy set up through the modern maternity system. To understand how this impacts women today, we must take a trip down the laneways of the various waves of feminism and understand the impact on maternity practices and beliefs.

I've said it, the sometime threatening and loaded word, "feminism." I am proud to be a midwife and I am proud to be a feminist researcher. I entered feminist research with trepidation and fear but then I read and now understand the importance of conducting research through a feminist lens. A highlight for me was when I was cited in a research paper as a "feminist researcher." I used feminist methodology in both my master's honours and PhD research. For my PhD, I used critical feminist theory.

As Bell Hooks wrote, feminism is for everybody (Hooks, 2000) and I believe that feminism aims for equality for all through identifying the constructs that make equality unachievable for women of all colours and individuals from marginalised groups. It is not man-hating or trying to replace men with women but identifying that the playing field is in no way level and actively working on ways to mobilise everyone on to the playing field and providing support for those that need it to be there.

The following explanations are simplistic and feminist scholars will pick me up on this, but I wanted to give a broad presentation on the waves of feminism and the impact on maternity care. The term "waves" is commonly used to describe the history of feminism, but this can be misleading, as many of the events occurred alongside or overlapping another wave.

Feminism and Birth

The First Wave

The first wave of feminism is remembered for the fight of the suffragettes in securing voting rights alongside other laws, such as marital and property rights in the Western world. New Zealand granted women the right to vote in 1893. In Australia, white women received the right to vote in 1902, the UK in 1918 (for over 30 years and if they or their husband had property), and the USA in 1920, the 19th Amendment to the Constitution was ratified to include women's right to vote.

Changes were also occurring in maternity practices. The attitude to labour pain changed from functional to pathological (Fannin, 2019). In a fascinating historical study of literature from New York in the early 1900s, Johnson and Quinlan (2015) demonstrate how midwives were becoming regulated and legislated alongside smear campaigns fuelled by physicians. Midwives sphere of practice legally became limited to "natural" births and any necessity for medicine or instruments became the legal domain of obstetricians (Yam, 2020). Obstetricians promoted birth in a controlled, hospital setting and middle and upper class women were lured with the promise of medicinal pain relief for a fee (Johnson & Quinlan, 2015). Obstetricians experimented with a range of medications under the belief that it was their duty to relieve pain. The long-term outcomes for women and babies were unclear and experimental medications included paraldehyde, rectal ether in oil, phenobarbital, chloroform, potassium bromide, cocaine, heroin, bromethyl, nitrous oxide, and scopolamine (called twilight sleep) (Eley et al., 2015; Johnson & Quinlan, 2015).

The introduction of twilight sleep originated from Germany and was known as the "Freiburg Method" (Johnson & Quinlan, 2015). The pharmacological combination of scopolamine and morphine injected intramuscularly produced an amnestic state, where the woman was not fully conscious, more pliant, and had no memory of the pain and experience of childbirth. Management of twilight sleep involved frequent memory tests and observation of behaviour in case of full unconsciousness or combative delirium and was performed in specific hospital settings.

Initially there was hesitancy from obstetricians on the use of twilight sleep and the popularity was because women campaigned for it, many from the suffragette movement (Barnett, 2005; MacIvor Thompson, 2019). In the USA, supporters of the use of twilight sleep set up the Twilight Sleep Association, which organised public campaigns through meetings, and newspaper and magazine articles written by women who experienced or witnessed twilight sleep. Magazine articles pushed the rhetoric of "painless childbirth," and used pictures of immaculate women and babies. Authors adopted the use of technical language to describe the use of twilight sleep and to give women knowledge to ask for this procedure from their doctors. Doctors were not keen on female writers demonstrating intelligence through understanding technical terms and procedures, yet the pro-twilight sleep campaign worked, and it was used throughout the early 1900s to the 1960s across high-resourced countries, including the USA, UK, and Australia (Barnett, 2005; Eley et al., 2015; Hairston, 1996). Inadvertently, the first wave of white middle- and upper-class feminists had a role in moving women away from female midwifery care at home to male obstetric care in hospitals, on beds and in stirrups (Johnson & Quinlan, 2015).

The Second Wave

The second wave of feminism arose from the activist movements during the 1960s with the classic book, *The Feminine Mystique* by Betty Freidan. In this book, based on 200 open-ended questions with her college classmates 15 years since graduation in the USA, Betty Freidan explored the despair and depression experienced by women in post-war suburban households. Although educated through high school and potentially college, starting careers, and working, white middle- and upper- class women were marrying, having families, and devoting to full-time housewife duties. The women she interviewed shared an emptiness and despondency of their situation, what Freidan identified as "the problem that has no name." As one of her interviewees described,

> *If you knock on any of these doors, how many women would you find whose abilities are being used? You'd find them drinking or sitting around talking to other women and watching children play because they can't bear to be alone, or watching TV or reading a book. Society hasn't caught up with women yet, hasn't found a way yet to use the skills and energies of women except to bear children. Over the last fifteen years, I think women have been running away from themselves. The reason the young ones have swallowed this feminine business is because they think if they go back and look for all their satisfaction in the home, it will be easier. But it won't be. Somewhere along the line a woman, if she is going to come to terms with herself, has to find herself as a person* (Friedan, 1963, p. 404).

The recognised frustration of women in suburban homes grew with letters of support (and hate) arriving at Freidan's home and developed into the creation of the National Organization for Women (NOW) to address the:

> ... *unfinished business of equality: equal opportunity for jobs and education, the right to abortion and child-care centers, the right to our own share of political power. It would unite women again in serious action* (Freidan, 2021, p. 456).

Many advancements were made, yet many were stalled, such as the Equal Rights Amendment (ERA), and backlash was felt from religious organisations and conservative factions (Nachescu, 2009). A movement had been created and women were able to challenge the perceived expectations of settling into the role of housewife alone.

By the beginning of the second wave, most women in high-resourced countries were birthing in hospitals managed by obstetricians. In opposition to the advancing medicalisation of birth, women wished to take back control and embraced a natural birth movement, one where women were aware of their birthing experience (not in an amnesic and sedated state) and learnt distraction and breathing techniques to cope with labour.

The impact of this was beginning to be felt, and activists and feminist scholars were starting to take notice. In the UK, the anthropologist Sheila Kitzinger was involved in the beginnings of the National Childbirth Trust and published her first book *The Experience of Childbirth* in 1962, based on her own homebirths, her observations as an anthropologist, and the teachings of Grantly Dick-Read and Lamaze (Kitzinger, 2015). In the USA, a collective of women published the infamous *Our Bodies, Our Selves*, which included a chapter on pregnancy and birth (Boston Women's Health Collective, 1971). This book has undergone nine editions, the most recent in 2011. The chapter starts with this explanation:

> *The purpose of this paper is to explain to women the experience of childbirth and the ideas and techniques of prepared childbirth from a women's liberation viewpoint. It is important that prepared childbirth be discussed in the context of a course on women and their bodies that includes sections on sexuality, anatomy, medical institutions, etc. My larger aim is to re-unite women's minds and bodies, not just for the brief period of childbirth, out in an overall program of overcoming our mental and physical oppression as women* (Boston Women's Health Collective, 1971, p. 127)

These and other texts explored breathing and distraction therapies alongside education to give women their power in birth back. It was a growing movement but not always a popular one due to the power of belief in patriarchal obstetrics.

Yet obstetric power remained throughout the 1970s and 1980s. The impact of obstetric management continued to be questioned, considering the evidence of rising caesarean rates. In 1993, Ann Oakley published her book *Essays on Women, Medicine, and Health*, where she asked:

> *What does it do to women to have their babies gestated and born so very much within such a closed structure of medical surveillance? It is hard to feel in control of one's body and one's destiny during sixteen trips to the hospital antenatal clinic for the ritual laying-on of hands by a succession of different doctors, none of them especially trained in the art of talking to the faces beyond the abdomens, or in the science of knowing about the interaction between mind and body, the connection between peace of mind and a competent cervix, or between emotional confidence and a coordinated uterus. What we see involved here are issues of control and responsibility that come up again and again in looking at women's health* (Oakley, 1993, pp. 12-13).

Ann Oakley identified how the dominant position of obstetricians resulted in the paternalistic belief that pregnancy and childbirth was a pathological process with the focus on the end product of the baby (Oakley, 1993). Brigitte Jordan named this "authoritative knowledge," which she described as:

> *... the knowledge that within a community is considered legitimate, consequential, official, worthy of discussion and appropriate for justifying particular actions by people engaged in accomplishing the tasks at hand* (Jordan, 1997, p. 58).

Basically, the popular belief from both within hospitals and in the community at large was that the medical establishment was right and safe, and the "at least you have a healthy baby" attitude prevailed. How women felt about their birthing experience was not seen as important or addressed as the woman didn't hold any useful knowledge and it was of no consequence (Jordan, 1997).

American anthropologist Robbie Davis-Floyd named the medicalised obstetric model of care "the technocratic model of birth," which she described as:

> *In accordance with this metaphor, a woman's reproductive tract is treated like a birthing machine by skilled technicians working under semi-flexible timetables to meet production and quality control demands ... The hospital itself is a highly sophisticated technological factory (the more technology the hospital has to offer, the better it is considered to be). As an institution it constitutes a more significant social unit than the individual or the family, so the birth process should conform more to institutional than personal needs... Through these procedures the natural process of birth is deconstructed into identifiable segments, then reconstructed as a mechanical process. Birth is thereby made to appear as though it confirms, instead of challenges, the technocratic model of reality upon which our society is based* (Davis-Floyd, 1993, pp. 278, 280, 281).

This could have been written today instead of 28 years ago. Policies and guidelines are written and developed by the colleges and hospitals that govern the practice. Women are expected to follow them and not have individual wishes. The mainstream obstetric management of pregnancy and birth hasn't changed dramatically in that time. What has increased is the caesarean rate.

Third Wave

The third wave of feminism was a wakeup call for second wave feminists. What was being noticed by women of colour, women with a disability, and women from the LGBTQI+ community was their lack of representation and voice in the second wave of feminism. Most feminist leaders and researchers had been white middle- and upper-class women speaking for white middle- and upper-class women. There was little recognition of the impact of being a woman and being black, disabled, and/or being from the LGBTI community. Emerging from the 1990s and Generation X in the USA, and a decade later in the UK and Australia, third wave feminists separated from the universality of experience from the second wave to identifying, accepting, and embracing the differences of women

(Aune & Holyoak, 2018; Pinterics, 2001). Boundaries were pushed in the third wave and women were challenged to be aware of their oppressions but also their privileges. Third wave feminists developed alongside the ascent of the internet and mass media (Snyder, 2008).

Third wave feminists tended to have a variety of attitudes to childbirth. Many disregarded the alternative birth movement and the hallowed achievement of a natural pain medication-free birth and argued that the technological view of birth could be beneficial for women (Beckett, 2005). Others identified the harm and picketed to keep birth centres and midwifery models of care open. No doubt the echo chambers of social media grow on the rhetoric of these dichotomised groups through being exposed to the views and images of the groups and individuals they follow. In that way, the authoritative knowledge of the chosen groups and views are continuously reinforced on the social media feed and opposing views silenced with a tap of the unfollow option.

Reproductive Justice

An essential maternity development from the third wave of feminism is reproductive justice. The reproductive justice framework was created by twelve black women who met in Chicago in 1994 at a pro-choice conference advocating for health reform and formed the Women of African Descent for Reproductive Justice group (Ross & Solinger, 2017). Through sharing their individual stories, the women focused on the entire reproductive journey and realised that abortion rights were one part of the longer journey but entwined throughout the reproductive journey was access to healthcare, poverty, education, jobs, and child-care. The combination of the following equation made up reproduction justice: reproduction rights + social justice = reproductive justice (Ross & Solinger, 2017).

There are three primary values to reproductive justice.

> *... (1) the right not to have a child; (2) the right to have a child; and (3) the right to parent children in safe and healthy environments. In addition, reproductive justice demands sexual autonomy and gender freedom for every human being* (Ross & Solinger, 2017, p. 65).

The movement expanded and in collaboration with other women's groups, they organized the largest protest in U.S. history at the time, with 1.15 million women and men at the March for Women's Lives in Washington April 25th, 2004.

The key to reproductive justice is identifying how oppressions of the past both controlled and shaped the reproductive rights of women of colour, First Nations, and migrant women in the current age. Both historical and current governmental health policies have deliberately impacted women's reproductive rights, which are noticeably different to white women. For example, population control during the time of European settlement, including slavery, outlawing intermarriage, and the Indian Removal Act. Post-Civil War, as white women were able to access contraception for a fee, African American women experienced poverty and violence in the South, First Nations women were having their children removed and sent to boarding schools, and wives of Chinese migrant men were prevented from immigrating to the U.S.

Historically, black women have experienced persecution in the field of obstetrics and gynaecology. From the use of enslaved black women to develop the surgical technique of repairing fistulas in the mid 1800's (Simms, 1886) through to the 1970's where hysterectomies were still performed for obstetric training purposes without the true informed consent of the women (Ross & Solinger, 2017).

The introduction of eugenics at the beginning of the 20th century promoted inhibiting the reproduction of persons based on race, ethnicity, religion, and disability, which could include forced sterilization. During the Civil Rights era of the 1960s, programs of coercive sterilization were established that targeted First Nations women, African American women, and Puerto Rican and Mexican immigrants. There were even recent allegations of forced sterilizations in U.S. immigration detention centres (Amiri, 2020). Meanwhile, throughout the 1960's and 70's, white women were discouraged from sterilization until she had fulfilled her reproducing role and with the permission of two doctors and a psychiatrist (Ross & Solinger, 2017).

Therefore, as Ross and Solinger (2017) summarises:

> *Not surprisingly, in the 1990s, after generations of sexuality- and fertility-related degradations—from slavery times throughout the twentieth century—a number of women of color spoke out together, making the case that their route to reproductive dignity did not depend on simply making good personal choices ...The women of color activists also pointed out that "choice," as conceived by white feminists, focused almost entirely on a woman's ability to prevent conception and motherhood. The activists, again pointing to their own history, objected to this singular focus on prevention...Once more drawing from the histories of their peoples, their families, and their communities, reproductive justice activists maintained that reproductive safety and dignity depended on having the resources to get good medical care and decent housing, to have a job that paid a living wage, to live without police harassment, to live free of racism in a physically healthy environment—all of these (and other) conditions of life were fundamental conditions for reproductive dignity and safety—reproductive justice—along with legal contraception and abortion* (Ross & Solinger, 2017, pp. 54,55,56).

Much of this history was played out in other colonised countries, such as Australia and Canada, especially regarding the treatment of First Nations women. In Australia, Aboriginal women experienced sexual abuse and exploitation on reserves and missions, had their children removed, experienced forced sterilisation, and were forced into domestic slavery (Andrews, 1996; Behrendt, 1993). In recent times, there were higher rates of out of home care of children, deaths in custody, and disproportionate rates of incarceration (Funston & Herring, 2016; Geia et al., 2020; Wilson et al., 2017).

The impact of racist policies and actions are evident in the appalling maternal statistics for women of colour and First Nations women today. In the UK, Asian women are twice as likely and black women five times as likely to die in childbirth compared to white British women (Womersley et al., 2021). In the USA, black women are 3-4 times more likely than white women to die in hospital, and both black and Hispanic women have higher caesarean rates (Oparah et al., 2018; Tangel et al., 2019). Preterm birth rates are higher in black women in the U. S. and

First Nations women in Australia compared to white women (Desisto et al., 2018; Kildea et al., 2019). Racial bias also impacts VBAC. Studies suggest that more African American women than white women plan a VBAC but have a repeat caesarean and experience underlying systemic racism (Miller & Baker, 2021).

The reproductive justice framework provides avenues for action and there are many services and programs that exist and continue to develop. An important consideration is the greater need for black, minority, and First Nations midwives, doulas, and healthcare professionals. In the USA, the National Association to Advance Black Birth (https://thenaabb.org) is a non-profit organisation advocating for black women and providing scholarships to support black midwifery students, and have developed a Black Birthing Bill of Rights to support women and to inform healthcare providers (NAABB, 2020). In Australia, the Rhodanthe Lipsett Indigenous Midwifery Charitable Fund (http://indigenousmidwives.org.au) provides scholarships and awards to "support and encourage Aboriginal or Torres Strait Islander people to undertake midwifery education and to expand their skills in caring for Indigenous mothers and their infants."

The focus on midwifery is deliberate. Midwifery is, by nature, a feminist profession. The traditional role of midwife is recognised in ancient scriptures, and traditional cultures had recognised midwifery roles in their societies. Midwife translates to "with woman" and there are many benefits to having midwifery care, which will be explored further in Chapter 6.

So, what does all the information above about the waves of feminism and reproductive justice have to do with having control? It is important for you to understand how the current maternity system is set up to make it difficult for women to have control. Being mindful of the shift from midwifery to obstetric care in hospital, to who holds the authoritative knowledge of birth and how systemic racism continues to disempower and disenfranchise women of colour give the bigger picture of control and power in maternal care. Understanding how the historical patriarchal systems are currently impacting women accessing maternity care helps us to understand how challenging it is for women to just say no to interventions. Saying no when you are at the bottom of the hierarchical ladder and being treated as if your wishes and concerns don't matter is not an easy option.

Women who say no or choose the alternate, non-mainstream maternity options (such as planning a VBAC) are seen as renegades and difficult. I have often been a renegade and it isn't easy. As a midwife, I experienced bullying and it took me to dark and troubling places, but it didn't change my renegade stance on giving women choice and respect. In my research, 51% of women in standard, fragmented maternity care were subject to hurtful comments that consisted of coercion and threats, just because they were planning a VBAC (Keedle et al., 2020).

I do believe that there are actions and preparation you can do to increase your feelings of control when pregnant after a previous caesarean. The four factors work together and synchronously, meaning that if you work on making the relationship factor better that will, in turn, help you feel more in control.

Being aware of what you wish for and how important that is to you is part of the control process. One of the essential steps to achieve this is to create a birth plan but I don't feel that all methods of birth planning are useful. In this next section, I will briefly discuss the research on birth plans and offer you a practice that I learnt when planning a VBAC which I used alongside the many women and their support teams I cared for as a midwife.

Birth Plans

The second wave feminist, childbirth educator, and anthropologist Shelia Kitzinger in the UK and Penny Simkin in the USA created the concept of the birth plan in the early 1980s (Kitzinger, 1992, 2015). The birth plan concept aimed to increase the trust and cooperation between women and health care professionals through the creation during pregnancy and alongside antenatal education, which would then be referred to during labour and birth (Kitzinger, 1992; Leap & Hunter, 2016).

Modern birth plans have a variety of designs including tick lists and online versions that are customisable. The World Health Organization recognises the benefit of using birth plans in improving maternal and newborn health (WHO, 2009). In the VBAC survey part of my PhD, 75% of respondents developed a birth plan. When asked if their healthcare provider supported the birth plan, more women who had midwifery continuity of care responded positively (75%) than if they saw a doctor (55%) or had standard antenatal care (35%). Obviously, if you are going to create a birth plan, you want your healthcare provider to support it, and there are some practical ways that I will explore to help you create a birth plan that helps you feel more in control, however the birth works out, and will gain the best support from your healthcare provider from a midwife's perspective.

There are a few ways to create your birth plan. Below, we hear from PhD candidate Catherine Bell, who has developed The Birth Map and trains doulas and midwives in her Birth Cartographer training.

Birth Mapping for Birth after Caesarean – Catherine Bell

A *Birth Map* is created through the process of Birth Cartography®. *Cartography is the art of making and using maps.* Birth Cartography, or Birth Mapping, is a process of careful and well-researched birth preparations, allowing you to make informed decisions about your care. These decisions are then documented in your Birth Map.

This process helps us explore not just the physical aspects, but also the political, emotional, and social aspects that influence our options.

Birth Mapping was a serendipitous creation, born out of frustrations with birth plans. Birth plans were falling short: some critical aspects missing, which stemmed from the language. The word *plan* was preventing conversations; people would say "plans get thrown out the window." Suggestions of *wishes* and *preferences* were reducing women's input into their own experience, were too easily dismissed and not always realistic.

The term *Map*, however, opened conversations. Maps have different pathways, and a journey is prepared for based on the possibility that detours may be needed. Instead of wishes and preferences, the focus is on *Informed Decisions.* The actual decisions are made during the journey, but advanced consideration allows for a less stressful and more aware process. This is reassuring for women, their partners, and the care providers.

Key to the process of Birth Cartography is that women are given the means of informed decision making: The Questions. *The Birth Map* was written to provide the questions that women need to start the conversations they need to have. Some women will only ask a few questions, others will need to ask more, and some may choose to ask none. What matters is that the woman can determine for herself which questions she needs to ask for her own journey and build a more realistic understanding of what birth can look like with her chosen care provider in her unique circumstances. The book is designed to give women the *opportunity* to explore their options on their own and is linked to a free independent online resource (https://birthmap.life), which has research articles and links to evidenced-based resources.

This process is focused on encouraging communication with the care provider and creating an "if this, then that" understanding of various pathways.

As a communication and decision-making process, Birth Mapping is intended to be adaptable to all those preparing for birth, as this approach will contextualise the individual and focuses on communication with the care provider.

When preparing for the birth after caesarean, the birth mapping process begins with understanding previous experience, considering our goals and motivations for the next birth, and placing this into the context of our current circumstances.

Birth Mapping breaks caesarean into four different types, with each type having different considerations:

1. The before-labour non-emergency, where the reasons for the caesarean are known and the timing is known well in advance. This may include an opportunity for a maternal-assisted caesarean, depending on our circumstances and the skill of the surgeon. If separation from the baby is required, we are ready for this and have in place a support system.
2. The before-labour emergency, where circumstances change suddenly, and a surgical birth may be critical. This can be a frightening time, having a preparation for this scenario helps ease stress. Preparations may be setting up a support system, understanding what this will look like, and who might be involved.
3. The after-labour non-emergency, where the woman may request a caesarean after labour has begun, or the caesarean is planned but labour begins first, or the woman accepts an offer of a caesarean after labour has begun.
4. The after-labour emergency caesarean, where circumstances have changed suddenly, exhaustion is evident, or a situation has arisen, and the surgical birth is recommended. It helps to ease stress by a preparation for this scenario.

If our expected pathway is a VBAC, we firstly choose a care provider that aligns with this goal. We build a support team that understands this goal and what role they will play. For the vaginal birth pathway, we have two possibilities: a spontaneous start or an induced start. Here we weigh up the risks, benefits, and timing. This decision will involve more than just a consideration of induction versus spontaneous. It will include practical considerations, such as personal history, distance to the hospital, hospital policies, support for before, during and after labour and birth, and the various *what ifs*. What if labour starts before 37 weeks? Or after 41 weeks? If the intention is to have an induction, what if labour begins before induction? This will be influenced by the reason for induction.

If we experienced labour previously, we may have clear ideas on what we need. If not, we may need to have a few more tricks up our sleeves. Independent childbirth education is a great way to learn techniques for labour and to help prepare our support person for this journey. We can then shape an order of business, which might include the different techniques we will try and what we will do if they are not working.

We will consider both non-medical and medical options, including the epidural. The medical procedures available to us require consent, from vaginal exams to epidurals, and this means we need to be able to make an informed decision. To this, we need to understand the risks and benefits, and alternatives to each procedure. This means an understanding of not just the procedure itself, but the impact it will have on our experience. For example, with the epidural, it may offer us pain relief, but also has some immediate and long-term risks. An epidural also means we will need a catheter inserted to drain our bladder and a drip inserted for hydration. If we have not had Syntocinon, we may also receive another drip with this labour augmenting drug. Each of these additional aspects needs to be considered as part of this decision. Given that an epidural increases the likelihood of an assisted delivery, which is associated with an increase in severe perineal trauma, many women like to avoid an epidural. However, it is helpful to ask ourselves, "under what conditions would I accept an epidural?"

For some, this is the turning point for them, and they would choose a caesarean, content with having experienced labour and feeling more comfortable with an in-labour non-emergency caesarean. They would be accepting the epidural in preparation for the caesarean. For others, they may have a personal time limit, or will base this decision on how they feel in the moment. Some will be comfortable with continuing along the vaginal pathway. There is no one way, and only you can determine what is right for you.

Catherine Bell

The Three Scenarios Exercise

In this section I will describe the method I have used for myself, in classes and with clients. The idea is inspired from the excellent book, *Birthing from Within* (England & Horowitz, 1998), which I was gifted during my first pregnancy. On a night shift where I was working alone in a children's ward, I gathered any pens I could find and plain paper and set about to do this exercise. The thing is, I can't now find this actual exercise in the book. I see something a little similar but not exactly it. That is why I say it is inspired by the activities in the book. The type of night shift, alert for buzzers, monitors, and cries, fuzzy pregnant-brain inspired. It was useful for me, and I stuck with my weird version throughout my practice with good feedback from clients, so whatever my brain did to alter what I was reading on that night shift, I'll own it and stick with it.

I did the practice alone, but when I started using this with clients and their support partners, I saw a vital part of the exercise, which is all about individual expectations and fears. I strongly recommend you do this with your support partner, the one who will be with you during labour and birth. This might be the same person who was there during your previous labour and caesarean, or they may be someone different. That doesn't matter. What matters is that you are both separately thinking about the next labour and birth and then coming together to have an exercise in communication.

Let's get started.

1. **Gather your supplies:** You don't need much here. It can be done with 1 pen and 3 pieces of paper, but if you have coloured pencils, crayons, or pens, then go and raid your child's art materials.

2. **Gather your support person:** You will both do the drawings at the same time but away from each other so you can't see what the other is drawing. Go to separate rooms or part of your home if you can.

3. **If you are alone:** That is completely okay. Some partners may not feel comfortable doing this and some don't have partners. You can do this alone. I did.

4. **Label each piece of paper:** On the top of each piece of paper, write the following titles

    » My ideal birth

    » My worst-case birth

    » My worst-case-made-better birth

5. **Get drawing:** Let your mind and imagination go with this. You can use stick figures or create an art gallery-worthy masterpiece. It's what ends up on the page that matters. I did stick figures. When you are drawing the ideal birth, think, "how do I want that birth to look?" It can be difficult to draw the worst-case birth, but I encourage you to face your fears and then draw them anyway. What does your worst-case birth look like? Finally, draw the worst-case birth made better. If you had that worst-case birth you drew, what could it look like to make the experience better?

6. **Instructions for support people:** Although this isn't your birthing experience, you have been chosen to be the support at the labour and birth. That is an honour that should be taken with reverence, but you must be aware that your previous experiences and your dreams also matter. With the ideal birth, draw how you would like to see this birthing experience be from your perspective. For your worst-case birth, you may have previous experience that you can draw on, even if you don't think about the worst-case birthing experience from your perspective. There is no right or wrong here, and I give you permission to go to dark places. It is only for a while and then the rainbow will shine through. For your worst-case-made-better, what do you think would make that worst-case scenario better?

7. **Take your time:** This doesn't need to be rushed but I think it is best to do in one sitting. Pour yourself a beverage. Take some deep breaths. Don't overthink it. Just go with the flow.

8. **Come together:** When you have both finished, come together. Be mindful and say to each other that you are sharing without

judgement, that there is no right or wrong, or competition; just sharing and listening. Take time to go through each scenario and listen to each other as you both explain what has been drawn. Be kind when sharing and talking about the worst-case scenario. You are both bringing your previous experiences and emotions to the surface. Be gentle, have tissues handy, and hold that space. If you need space at this time, recognise that but come back to the exercise, as it isn't complete. Really listen to each other on the worst-case scenario made better. I would often see real connection and growth at this point, as different people would put down different images and to make things better. These are little rainbows shining from the page.

9. **Review on your own:** If you did this alone, then spend some time looking at your drawings and thinking about the meaning behind them. You might want to share them with a trusted friend, relative, or your healthcare provider if you feel that you trust them with these important insights.

10. **Create your birth plans—Plan A and plan B:** You can take a break and come back to this, but you can now transform those pictures into two birth plans. You can call these whatever you wish; you are the creator here. They might be plans or preferences. The two you will create will be for your ideal birth or plan A and your worst-case-made-better plan or plan B. Start with plan A. Look at the ideal birth picture of yours and your support persons (if done). What are in the pictures that you can now put in words? I'm not going to prompt, as in my experience, they all look so different. You might have the location, people present, methods for coping in labour, or music. Write these down. This plan A is individual to you (and your support person).

    Plan B is important. If you did have your worst case or similar, what was present in the drawings of the worst case made better that are important to you (and your support person)? Write these down. These are your ways of keeping control when the situation isn't what you had planned for.

11. **Present and discuss these with your midwife/doctor:** Once you have your two lists and you have discussed these with your support person or team, present them and discuss them with your midwife or doctor if you feel comfortable. I hope you do have that relationship that is open to talking about your plans. They can be empowering for your healthcare team too. There is a recognition from them that you have thought about your plan A but that you have also thought about your plan B. In my experience, when I have had been with women where we needed to use plan B, and I have discussed this with other healthcare professionals, they have gone out of their way to accommodate the plan B list as much as they can. Midwives and doctors do genuinely care, and if they have some goals that are achievable in a difficult situation, they will usually help them be achieved. That is why it is important that the healthcare team are aware of your plan A and plan B.
12. **Reflect on your birth experience:** What type of birth did you end up having? Plan A, plan B, or a combination? We will explore this further on in the book.

Three Scenario Examples

I was honoured to be the midwife to the amazing Sasha and her partner Brian. We journeyed through two pregnancies and births together and have remained in contact. Sasha's full story is available in Chapter 10. We did the three-scenario exercise for her first planned VBAC and they have kindly given me permission to share them here.

Brian's drawings

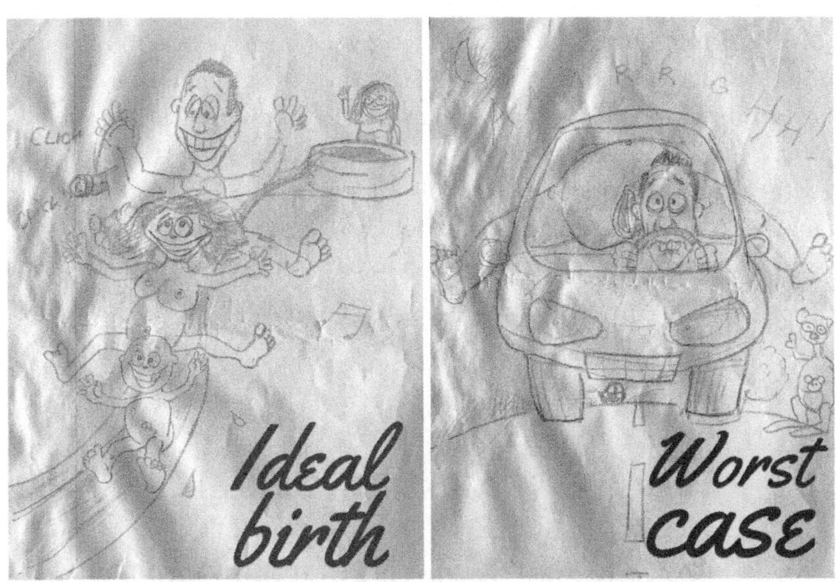

Sasha's drawings

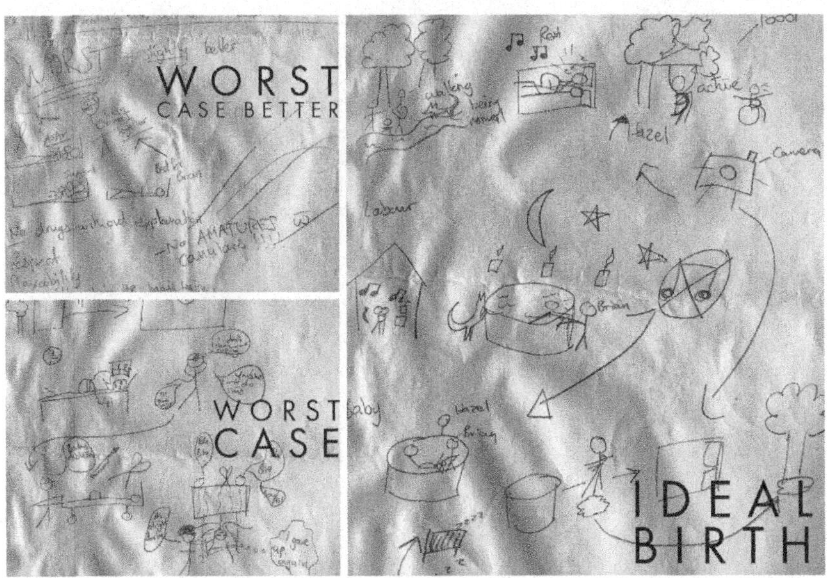

Summary

In this "having control" chapter, I have given you a history of feminism and reproductive justice to explain how the current maternity system makes it difficult for women to feel in control of their wishes and birth options. I then moved on to look at the importance of birth plans and how they can help you look at what is important in a variety of birthing scenarios and how in turn they can help you feel more in control of your birthing decisions. We will now move onto looking at the importance of having confidence.

HAVING CONTROL CHECKLIST

- ☑ **Recognise the role of feminism and reproductive justice on the current maternity system**
- ☑ **Create a birth plan**
- ☑ **Discuss your birth plan with your midwife / doctor**

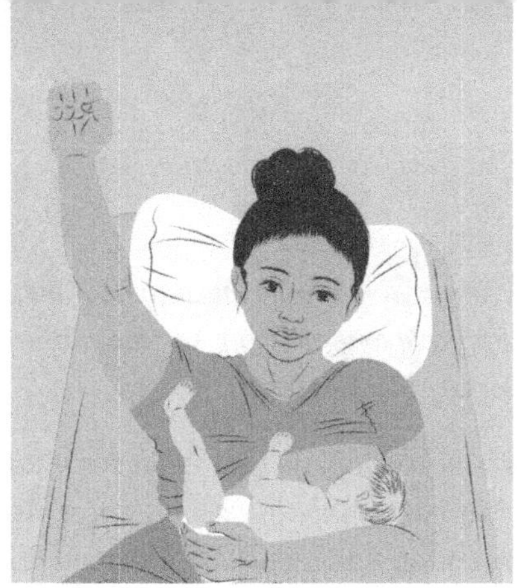

Chapter 6

HAVING CONFIDENCE

Why is Confidence Important?

In the four factors, "having confidence" is described as you having confidence in your ability to have the birth you want. It sounds simplistic but if you, for example, are planning a VBAC and you haven't had a vaginal birth before, then having confidence that you can have a VBAC isn't always easy to come by. This lack of confidence may have been reinforced by the negative language used during your caesarean experience. You may have been told that you needed to be induced, as you "failed" to go into labour naturally and then you may have "failed" to progress or be told you were a "failed" induction. You may have been told your pelvis was too small or misshapen or that your baby didn't fit through your pelvis. Firstly, don't believe it. It is more likely a failure to wait from the healthcare provider or guidelines than any failure on your part. Having a baby isn't a university exam. It's a rite of passage. You can't fail it, but you experience it.

Emili felt the impact of negative language following her first emergency caesarean. Her complete story is in Chapter 10.

> *When the time came, I went to hospital to be induced. After 36 hours of labour, I had to have emergency c-section, failure to progress, and pushing for too long.*
>
> *Being a first-time mum, I had no idea what went wrong and why my body failed me. My baby's safety was my top priority, so I felt like a failure. I was emotional, upset, and cried through the whole process.*

This negative language has a significant detrimental impact on our belief in our bodies and self-confidence. This is also something women are used to. We are constantly bombarded with images in the media and online that set out to identify our individual body failings. We are either too fat or too thin. Our breasts are too small, too large, misshapen, or missing. Our hair needs more conditioning. We need smoother legs without hair. Our lips aren't pouty enough. We don't wear enough or we wear too much makeup. The list could go on forever. We are bombarded by this rhetoric from a young age, and it just gets worse and worse.

Think about the language and media about ageing. Menopause is looked at with disdain, and wrinkles need to be obliterated until we have faces that are no longer able to express emotion. The constant pressure for perfection, which is a software-altered image, feeds into our mistrust and dissatisfaction with our bodies. Then you have a traumatic birth and absorb the negative language that, again, blames us and our bodies. No wonder we have no confidence that we can push babies out of our vaginas.

If this sounds familiar to you, then please don't despair. You *can* build up your confidence and the best way is to understand that knowledge is power. You are already building up your confidence by reading this book and gaining all the information so far.

How Can I Gain Confidence in My Body?

The suggestions that I will explore in this chapter focus on getting to know your body better, increasing knowledge about labour and birth, and seeking support from your peers.

Figure 1 - Increasing your confidence wheel

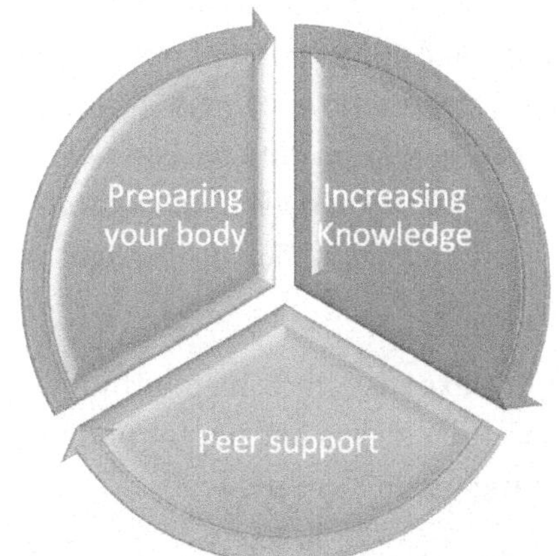

Preparing Your Body

In my master's honours study exploring women's experiences of planning a VBAC at home, there was a main theme of "it's never happening again," which was split into "why it's never happening again" and "how it's never happening again." The themes in "why" explored the previous caesarean and the reasons why the women did not want to repeat that experience. The themes under "how it's not happening again" explored the process, avenues, and activities that women did to prepare for a VBAC at home. I found that women prepared both mentally and physically for the birth, which included using relaxation and breathing techniques, and exercise. Below are some excerpts from the thesis where Carol identifies her relaxation methods and Natalie gives an overview of the health and exercise changes she adopted during her pregnancy.

> *I did a hypnobirthing course, which was really good. That helped with my breathing and just getting into the zone. I did some yoga. In bed, I would practice the breathing and listen to, you get a CD with the hypnobirthing book, listening to positive affirmations and things* (Carol) (Keedle, 2015, p. 150).

> *I saw a naturopath and started ... training, ... I got an exercise bike, and I was on the bike for 30 minutes a day and I didn't eat what the diabetes clinic told me to eat. I ate more of a naturopathic diet. I took apple cider vinegar. I stopped eating grains ... I got my calories from protein and stuff. I took a naturopathic diabetes tablet with chromium and cinnamon ... I cut out sugar, obviously, and started cooking with alternatives and I only put on 5 kilos in my pregnancy*" (Natalie) (Keedle, 2015, p. 151).

Kari enjoys running for exercise and she continued to run throughout her pregnancies. Kari's full story is in Chapter 10, but here is a snippet of her thoughts on running during pregnancy.

> *On the topic of running, after I ruptured, I questioned if I should have been running throughout that pregnancy and thought I had potentially put my baby at risk every time I ran. But then, the OB who assisted with the delivery and surgery said the fact that I ran so much was likely a contributing factor to why I had a good outcome given our birth situation. That comment is what pushed me through my weekly runs. I needed this for my and my baby's health. While I thoroughly enjoy running and love the self-challenge of running, my miles took me to new limits physically, mentally, and emotionally during this pregnancy. I'll never forget my last week of runs with her in my belly. Anticipating her arrival. Enjoying the time with me, her, the sun, and music. The time to be intentional and thoughtful of breathing through every step or Braxton Hicks contraction.*

There can be many benefits to continuing to exercise or to introduce exercise programs into your pregnancy. The Australian Pregnancy Care Clinical Practice Guidelines advise that "*usual physical activity during pregnancy has health benefits and is safe*" (Department of Health, 2020, p. 11.13). Benefits of physical activity or exercise during pregnancy include maintaining or improving cardiorespiratory fitness, lower weight gain, regulation of blood glucose for women with gestational diabetes, reducing the severity of lower back and pelvic musculoskeletal pain symptoms, and protecting against unplanned caesareans (Brown et al., 2020; Dipietro et al., 2019). It is suggested that women incorporate aerobic, strengthening, and pelvic floor exercises throughout pregnancy.

For further information on conditions or complications during pregnancy that can impact exercise and for suggestions on exercise types and healthy eating, please refer to the relevant website for your country.

» Australia - Raising Children network website:
https://raisingchildren.net.au/pregnancy/health-wellbeing/healthy-lifestyle/exercise-in-pregnancy-for-women

» USA – Centres for Disease Control and Prevention (CDC):
https://www.cdc.gov/physicalactivity/basics/pregnancy/index.htm

» UK – National Health Service (NHS):
https://www.nhs.uk/pregnancy/keeping-well/exercise/

Yoga

The practice of yoga has increased in popularity in the last decade. Zhang et al. (2021) found the prevalence of yoga tripled amongst adults in the USA from 2002 to 2017, with younger adults showing the highest increase. Yoga originated from ancient Indian practices and the Sanskrit translation of yoga is "to unite" or "to yoke," meaning that yogic practices lead to a harmony between the mind and the body, and the body and nature (Basavaraddi, 2015; Kwon et al., 2020).

The practice of yoga positions is one aspect (limb) of yoga philosophy. Yoga philosophy is divided into eight limbs, which are divided into three levels and can be depicted as the tree of yoga (Hayase & Shimada, 2018; Iyengar, 2013). The roots and trunk describe the ethical and moralistic principles of yoga philosophy. The branches and leaves relate to the yogic practices of *àsanas* (yoga positions) and *pràṇàyàma* (breathing) (Iyengar, 2013), which are the practices taught in yoga classes.

Yoga has been found to promote feelings of relaxation through modulating the autonomic nervous system (ANS) (Hayase & Shimada, 2018). The ANS controls body processes such as blood pressure, heart and breathing rates, digestion and metabolism, and is composed of the sympathetic and parasympathetic divisions of the nervous system (Low, 2020). While the sympathetic nervous system prepares the body for fight and flight through increasing heart rate and slowing digestion, the parasympathetic division conserves and restores through lowering heart rate, decreasing blood pressure, and stimulating digestion (Low, 2020).

A small Japanese study followed women through their pregnancy in two groups (Hayase & Shimada, 2018). The intervention group attended yoga classes once a week with optional at home yoga practice, and the control group didn't attend yoga classes. The women had their salivary α-amylase levels measured, which indicates the stress status of the sympathetic nervous system, alongside their perceived stress scores, their sleep log records, and heart rate variability. Hayase and Shimada (2018) found that participating in a yoga class significantly decreased salivary α-amylase levels compared to before-class levels, and that sleep time was longer in the yoga group. The results of this small study suggest that practicing yoga improved sleep and reduced stress in pregnant women (Hayase & Shimada, 2018), which supported previous studies on the immediate effects of yoga on stress in pregnancy (Kusaka et al., 2016).

A randomised control study from Iran found that women having their first baby, who attended a one-hour yoga class three times a week from 26 weeks gestation, had lower induction of labour and caesarean rates, as well as shorter duration of labour compared to the no-yoga group (Jahdi et al., 2017). Campbell and Nolan (2019) interviewed women who participated in yoga classes throughout their pregnancy. In the interviews conducted prior to starting yoga classes, the women were nervous and lacked confidence in thinking they can have the birth they wish for, including women who had a previous birth. Following attending yoga classes, women had gained confidence in their ability to manage labour and after the birthing experience, women were able to reflect on how practising yoga helped them during labour and birth (Campbell & Nolan, 2019).

> *I had been practising yoga and so therefore had built a relationship up with my body ... Having confidence in your body, because that's the most important thing: knowing that you can do it, believing that you can – Paula* (Campbell & Nolan, 2019, p. 79).

Similar findings were found in a qualitative study from Brazil which stated that women found practicing yoga increased their perception of self-confidence and self-esteem, alongside increased autonomy in managing their pregnancy (De Campos et al., 2020).

Practicing yoga during pregnancy can potentially decrease your stress levels, increase your quality of sleep, and build up your confidence in your body. If you are interested in practising yoga, please find a qualified yoga teacher in your area that teaches pregnancy yoga, as there are positions that need to be avoided during pregnancy.

Increasing Knowledge: Alternative Birthing Classes

There are many ways that you can increase your knowledge, from reading research to hearing women's stories. Many women who plan a VBAC have realised how the cascade of intervention impacted their labour journey to caesarean and wish to avoid or limit interventions in their subsequent labour. Interventions can include pharmacological pain relief, such as epidurals or morphine injections. If there is a plan to avoid this, then there should be a plan on learning about alternate methods to manage pain in labour. There is debate in some alternate birthing communities on whether to call contractions painful or use different terminology. Please feel free to use whatever terminology works for you but I won't lie and say you can make birth painless. Pain is defined by the International Association for the Study of Pain (2020) as:

> *An unpleasant sensory and emotional experience associated with, or resembling that associated with, actual or potential tissue damage* (Raja et al., 2020, p. 1977).

This definition doesn't really work for the sensation of pain in labour due to labour being a normal physiological process. A fascinating updated literature review on the nature of labour pain explored the experience of labour in published research (Whitburn et al., 2019). The authors challenged the current beliefs of many healthcare providers that depicts labour pain as suffering, and, therefore, a pathological process that should be managed with medication (Whitburn et al., 2019). This belief originated with the availability of pain relief and the move to hospital births, alongside the first wave of feminism, but is still prevalent across high resource countries today. The literature review concluded with these comments on the nature of labour pain:

> *Although incredibly intense and challenging, it is very different in nature to other typical pains. If a woman can sustain the belief that her pain is purposeful (i.e., her body working to birth her baby), if she interprets her pain as productive (i.e., taking her through a process to a desired goal) and the birthing environment is safe and supportive, it would be expected that she would experience the pain as a non-threatening, transformative life event. Changing the conceptualisation of labour pain to a purposeful and productive pain may be one step to improving women's experiences of it and reducing their need for pain interventions* (Whitburn et al., 2019, p. 34).

The question then moves to exploring the methods and techniques available for women to feel safe and supported and feel that labour pain is being productive. There are a variety of methods available, such as acupressure, massage, relaxation and breathing techniques, visualisations, yoga, and other complementary therapies.

There are also many courses, both online and face to face, that explore these methods, such as hypnobirthing, Calmbirth, SheBirths, and Lamaze, to name a few. There are also VBAC specific classes. In our VBAC survey, 30% of women accessed alternative therapy education classes (Keedle et al., 2020). In Chapter 8, having an active labour, I will go into more details about these classes.

Peer Support

Throughout the research I have done on VBAC, women have highlighted the importance of peer support. Most peer support has been in the form of online social media groups. These groups can be a source of education, support, encouragement, and advocacy for women who are planning a VBAC or a repeat caesarean, and I believe they can be helpful in boosting confidence. However, not all groups are upfront with their views and biases, and women can experience hostility and judgment when posting a concern or experience that other members in the group don't agree with.

I suggest having a good scroll and search of posts to ensure you are in the right supportive environment for your pregnancy and birthing decisions. Due to the number of available social media groups, I can't list them in this book, but I do encourage you to go online and find a tribe that will be of use and support you.

Not all support groups are on social media and if you are able to find one, two, or more individuals that can support you on your journey that you can meet up with virtually or face to face, then I encourage that too.

Reading and hearing experiences from women who have planned a birth after caesarean can increase your understanding and boost your confidence. There are women's stories in this book for you to read and identify with but also to inspire and give you confidence. You can also hear women's stories of birth after caesarean through different podcasts. Below are a few I know and recommend.

Podcasts

- VBAC Birth Stories: https://msha.ke/vbacbirthstories/
- The VBAC Homebirth Stories Podcast: https://themotherhoodcircle.com.au/podcast/
- The VBAC link Podcast: https://www.thevbaclink.com/podcast/
- VBAC Babes Podcast: https://linktr.ee/vbacbabes

Summary

In this chapter, we have explored the factor of "having confidence," which included preparing your body, increasing your knowledge, and seeking peer support. Although it can be challenging to feel confident about your ability to have the birth you wish, especially if you have had a previous traumatic birthing experience, the methods discussed in this chapter can help you gain more confidence and prepare you for the birth you are planning after caesarean. Another aspect of the "having confidence" factor that women highlighted in my PhD findings was the importance of feeling that their healthcare provider was also confident in their ability to have a VBAC. It was important for women to feel that their midwife or doctor believed in their ability to have a VBAC and that they were actively supporting them in achieving this birth experience. You want to have the right team beside you and supporting you, and this is what we will explore in the next chapter, "having a relationship."

HAVING CONFIDENCE CHECKLIST

- ☑ **Recognise how negative language may have impacted your confidence.**
- ☑ **Prepare your body with exercise and eating well.**
- ☑ **Increase your knowledge about tools to use during labour and birth.**
- ☑ **Find your peer support tribe and read/listen to women's stories.**

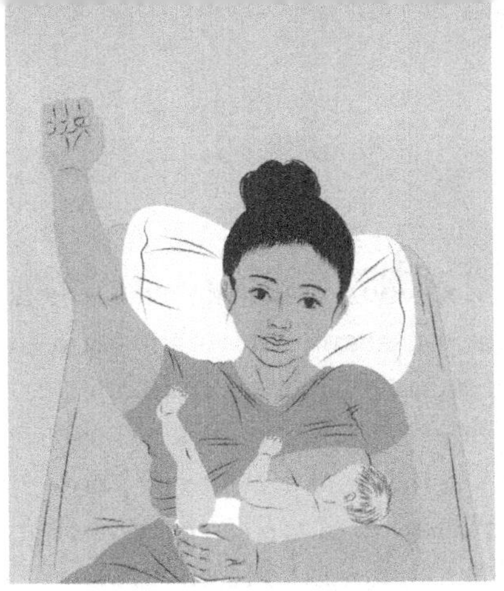

Chapter 7

HAVING A RELATIONSHIP

Choose Your Team

As I write this, the Paralympics is happening in Tokyo, and it makes me think of the strength and determination these elite athletes need to achieve their dreams to compete and to win a medal. No doubt, they met people along the way that said they couldn't do it, but they chose to continue and train hard to get a place on their national team. Most athletes will compete in one or two Olympic or Paralympic games, and they will remember these experiences for a lifetime.

The athletes needed a good support crew beside them providing support, expert advice, and encouragement. This support team, led by a coach, doesn't stand on the podium to receive the medals, and take the lime-light away from the athlete. They know when to step back and their joy and job satisfaction is seeing the accomplishment of the athlete.

I believe there are many parallels with birthing experiences. Women generally only have one or a few more births, and they remember the experiences for a lifetime. Women often put a lot of mental and physical preparation into the birthing experience and will come across a variety of opinions on their decisions, many not even asked for. Often, though, we don't think about our team. We might get a different healthcare provider at each pregnancy visit, or we go to one due to our health insurance status. We might even return to a healthcare provider that wasn't the most supportive last time but at least you know them. We might also be limited due to our location or resources. But what if we could choose our team and what if we chose the team based on how much support and encouragement they would give us?

As mentioned in Chapter 4, in the VBAC survey, over half of women in standard care received hurtful comments from a healthcare provider when planning a VBAC. These comments ranged from saying that parts of the woman's body were faulty to stating the woman or baby would die if they had a VBAC.

Imagine for a moment you were an elite track athlete racing in the 100m sprint with a spot on your national team, and then your coach said to you, "well, you could run the race, but you are putting yourself at great risk if you do. You could die from a cardiac arrest before you get to the finish line! Also, your legs are just too short and not made for running. I think it would be better for you to watch the race from your couch and stop planning this silly adventure. Let me make the decision for you, as I am the expert here." Would you want to continue with that coach, or would you go and find a coach that, instead, said "I believe in you. I will support you. I can see you on the podium with the gold medal! It won't be easy, and you will, at times, doubt yourself, but I will be there at every step of the way, encouraging you and giving you my expert knowledge. Remember, this is your body, your decision, and I respect and honour that." I think I would want the second coach.

Now, imagine that scenario but with your birthing team. "Well, you could plan a VBAC, but you are putting yourself at great risk if you do. You could die from a uterine rupture, or you could kill your baby! Also, your pelvis is just too narrow and not made for birthing. I think it would be better for you to book an elective caesarean and stop planning this silly adventure. Let me make the decision for you, as I am the expert here." Or "I believe in you. I will support you. I can see you holding your baby straight after your birth! It won't be easy, and you will, at times, doubt yourself, but I will be there at every step of the way, encouraging you and giving you my expert knowledge. Remember, this is your body, your decision, and I respect and honour that."

Some of the women who have shared their stories in this book have experienced hurtful comments from healthcare professionals. Here are some excerpts from the stories of Kari, Jordon, and Emili, where they describe these comments and experiences.

> *The first MFM [doctor] I saw didn't give any consideration to the research I had done, what I wanted from a future birth, how I felt, or what mattered to me. I was immediately dismissed. The short answer: why would you want this? You'll kill your baby and kill yourself. Honestly, there wasn't much of a long answer. Luke and I sat in a small exam room while three doctors stood over us lecturing us on why this should be dismissed. I barely made it out of the clinic without bursting into tears. That was an absolutely terrible appointment, and I won't forget how I was treated and felt. That car ride home was hard.* Kari

> *I went home after every appointment crying my eyes out after hearing on repeat, "Your previous c-section, previous big baby, and your high BMI mean you shouldn't try for a VBAC because you and your baby might die." At one stage, I recall her calling in the Register after I went off at her because she had told me in no uncertain terms that I was putting my baby at risk and was going to kill them.* Jordon

> *On every appointment, they would talk about risk of scar ruptures and brain damage, and asked questions like, "what will your husband say to your other kids if you die in labour? How would you feel knowing that you could have a normal, healthy baby and instead, got one with brain damage? Do you realise how would that change your family?"* Emili

In comparison to these hurtful experiences is Naomi's words about the team she had supporting her VBAC.

> *Being surrounded by support people that believed in me and supported me throughout my labour made me able to cope with it. The skills*

of the midwives to help the baby move lower and the willingness to support me, even though I did not have continuous monitoring and was not in a hospital, are the things that prevented me from having a repeat caesarean. Naomi

After analysing hundreds of hurtful comments, I know women are told comments like these frequently and they are based on exaggerated and unlikely facts. I would love more women to feel supported like Naomi, so let's explore how you can choose a team that will guide, support, and help you achieve the birth you want.

Different Models of Care

There is a variety of different maternity models of care that exist. I won't be able to discuss each type, but I will explore the main concepts, which are whether the model is continuity or fragmented and whether you see a midwife or doctor. Continuity of care means that you see the same midwife or doctor for each pregnancy appointment, they provide care or you during labour and birth, and they provide care for you during the post-birth period for up to 6 weeks.

Fragmented care means that you see a different midwife or doctor at each appointment, during labour and birth the midwife and/or doctor, you see are whoever is on shift and there are different healthcare professionals who attend you in the post-birth period. Most women experience fragmented care, and many don't know that continuity models are available.

Midwives are qualified and registered internationally recognised healthcare professionals who practice midwifery. Midwifery is defined by the International Confederation of Midwives (ICM, 2017) as:

> *... an approach to care of women and their newborn infants whereby midwives:*
>
> » *optimise the normal biological, psychological, social, and cultural processes of childbirth and early life of the newborn.*

- *work in partnership with women, respecting the individual circumstances and views of each woman*
- *promote women's personal capabilities to care for themselves and their families*
- *collaborate with midwives and other health professionals as necessary to provide holistic care that meets each woman's individual needs (ICM, 2017).*

Midwives can work privately, in groups, and in the public maternity care system. Obstetricians are medical doctors who have trained and specialised in the medical and surgical care of women. Obstetricians can work privately and in public hospitals. The maternity care system works well when midwives and doctors collaborate with each other when required, and there are many places where this occurs.

Midwifery continuity of care (CoC) is where the primary healthcare professional is a midwife who provides your pregnancy care, is on call for your labour and birth, and provides post-birth care for up to 6 weeks. There are many different terms for midwifery CoC dependent on your location. It can be called midwifery group practice, caseload, privately practicing midwives, and lead maternity carer. Obstetric CoC is where the primary healthcare professional is a doctor who provides your pregnancy care, on call for birth and limited postnatal care, and can be known as private obstetricians, OB-GYN, consultant, and other terms.

Research Around CoC

There has been much research on the benefits of midwifery CoC. The Cochrane Collaboration (https://www.cochranelibrary.com), which is an internationally recognised source of reviewing and publishing systematic reviews of randomised control trials, has published a review on midwifery CoC. In their review, they found 15 studies, which, in total, involved 17,674 women (Sandall et al., 2016). It concluded that:

> *The main benefits were that women who received midwife-led continuity of care were less likely to have an epidural. In addition, fewer women had episiotomies or instrumental births. Women's chances*

of a spontaneous vaginal birth were also increased and there was no difference in the number of caesarean births. Women were less likely to experience preterm birth, and they were also at a lower risk of losing their babies. In addition, women were more likely to be cared for in labour by midwives they already knew. The review identified no adverse effects compared with other models (Sandall et al., 2016, p. 2).

There has been some research on the benefits of midwifery CoC for women planning a VBAC. A small study from China compared women who had midwifery CoC to women who had standard care (Zhang & Liu, 2016). The group that had midwifery CoC had shorter labours, less postpartum haemorrhage rates, and higher VBAC rates of 88% compared to 68% in the standard care group (Zhang & Liu, 2016).

The quality of CoC is important, as the following study demonstrates. A recent study from Australia compared two similar models of care for women who had a previous caesarean (Homer et al., 2021). Both models offered CoC during pregnancy, but the models had teams of midwives, so women didn't always see the same midwife. One model offered CoC during labour and birth but as it was a team approach, women didn't always have a midwife they knew well. Women, in both models, reported seeing 4 to 6 midwives during their pregnancy for appointments and 69% of women wished they knew the midwife that attended them in labour, suggesting they didn't know the midwife. The study found no significant differences in VBAC rates between the two models, which is unsurprising, given the lack of actual continuity of care by the same midwife. The authors recognised that more studies are needed to compare midwifery continuity of care models where women see the same midwife (Homer et al., 2021).

Survey Results for Models of Care

In my PhD VBAC survey, we compared the experiences of women who had planned a VBAC and had accessed midwifery CoC, doctor CoC, and standard fragmented care. The findings I will discuss here are from the published paper, "Women's experiences of planning a vaginal birth after caesarean in different models of maternity care in Australia"

(Keedle et al., 2020). When we explored the factor relationship, we looked at a few different areas. These were:

» Appointment times

» Receiving positive support from midwife/doctor

» Receiving hurtful comments from midwife/doctor

» MADM & MORi scores

Appointment Times

Relationships take time to develop and maintain. In the survey, women identified the length of time, on average, their pregnancy appointments with their midwife or doctor were. The range was from 5 to 10 minutes, all the way to over 1 hour. The results can be seen in Figure 2. Most appointment times for women who had CoC with a doctor or had fragmented care was 10 to 15 minutes, followed by 15 to 20 minutes. For women who had midwifery CoC, most appointment times were 30 to 60 minutes, followed by 20 to 30 minutes. 22% of women who had CoC with a midwife had appointments that were over 1 hour, compared to 2% of fragmented care and 0% of CoC with a doctor.

As a midwife who has worked in midwifery CoC models, this makes a lot of sense to me. An appointment would mainly be at the woman's house and include at least one cup of tea. I can't drink hot tea in less than 15 minutes and find out how the woman and her family are going and then do the physical checks of blood pressure and abdominal palpation and listen to the baby.

Figure 2. Length of time for pregnancy appointments under different models of care (Keedle et al., 2020, p. 11).

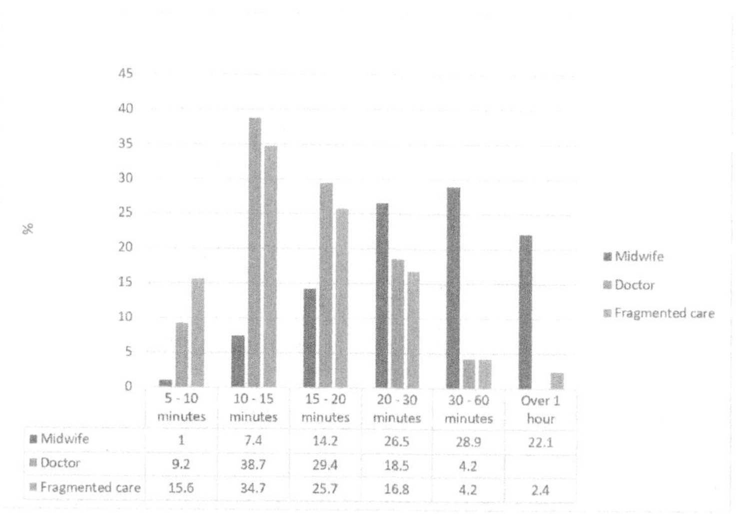

	5 - 10 minutes	10 - 15 minutes	15 - 20 minutes	20 - 30 minutes	30 - 60 minutes	Over 1 hour
Midwife	1	7.4	14.2	26.5	28.9	22.1
Doctor	9.2	38.7	29.4	18.5	4.2	
Fragmented care	15.6	34.7	25.7	16.8	4.2	2.4

Receiving Positive Support

As I mentioned at the beginning of this chapter, you deserve positive support from your midwife or doctor. In the VBAC survey, most women did receive positive support but there were statistically significant differences across models of care. For women who had midwifery CoC, 89.7% of women received positive support compared to 70.6% of women who had CoC with a doctor and 76.6% of women who had fragmented care.

Alongside positive support was whether women felt their midwife or doctor was confident in their ability to have a VBAC. There were significant differences here. Two questions were asked: one was if you thought your midwife/doctor was confident in your ability to have a VBAC while you were pregnant, and the other was during your labour. During pregnancy, 88.7% and during labour, 83.3% of women who had midwifery CoC felt their midwife was confident in their ability to have a VBAC compared to CoC with a doctor (70.6% during pregnancy and 61.3% during labour) and fragmented care (53.9% during pregnancy and 55.7% during labour). It is difficult to continue with your birthing wishes when you feel that the midwife or doctor has no confidence in your ability to achieve it, just like that coach who doesn't think you will make it to the finish line.

Receiving Hurtful Comments from Midwife or Doctor

As already discussed, most women received hurtful comments from healthcare professionals during their VBAC journey. Over half of women (51%) who had standard, fragmented care received hurtful comments compared to 35% of women who had midwifery CoC and 24% of women who had CoC. It is important to note here that the hurtful comment may not have come from the midwife or doctor, but could have come from a different healthcare provider they saw during their journey. For example, many women said they had to see a doctor when they were having midwifery CoC to approve their VBAC, and during that appointment, they received hurtful comments. In the next version of the survey, I will add a question to clarify who the hurtful comment came from.

MADM & MORi Scores

In the VBAC survey, we included two validated scales that were designed by researchers in Canada (https://www.birthplacelab.org). These were Mothers Autonomy in Decision Making scale (MADM) and Mothers on Respect Index (MORi). The MADM assesses the degree of autonomy in decision making women felt they were provided by midwives or doctors (Vedam et al., 2017a; Vedam et al., 2019) and in the survey, we used this to measure the factors "having control" and "having confidence." The higher the score the more involved women felt in the decision making for pregnancy and birth. In the VBAC survey, women who had midwifery CoC had statistically significant higher MADM scores than women who had CoC with a doctor or fragmented care.

The MORi measures respectful maternity care with higher scores, indicating more respectful interactions with midwives/doctors (Vedam et al., 2017b). In the VBAC survey, there were significantly higher MORi scores in women who had midwifery CoC, followed by

CoC with a doctor then fragmented care. This indicates that women felt they were treated with more respect in CoC models of care.

What is Good Support?

The results of the VBAC survey found that women who had CoC with a midwife were more likely to feel in control of their wishes and choices, feel more confident about their ability to have a VBAC, be more active in labour, and have a relationship based on equality and respect compared to women who had CoC with a doctor or had standard, fragmented care. This study also demonstrated that not all CoC models offer good support, as it compared midwifery CoC to CoC with a doctor. This study in no way means that you can't get fantastic care with a doctor and there are many obstetricians that provide great support for women planning a VBAC. But the statistics showed the difference in the models of care that favoured midwifery CoC.

During my master's honours study on women planning a homebirth after caesarean, I also conducted a focus group of privately practicing midwives. These are midwives in Australia that offer continuity of care as private midwives and most offer homebirth services. When I asked what they do differently when caring for women with a previous caesarean, they identified the importance of debriefing, and one midwife shared her thoughts in the quote below.

> *It's respect and partnership, you're not some superior person that has this knowledge that the woman doesn't have, she equally has knowledge of herself and her body and you're there just to provide information and talk that through with her, it's an equal partnership and just in the fact that you respect her and her choices, she wants to choose your care and she wants to birth at home and she is fully informed then we have the skills to support that* (Keedle, 2015, p. 146).

How to Find a Coc Model of Care

There are an increasing amount of midwifery continuity of care models becoming available for women and I suggest really exploring your local areas to see what is available to you. You can contact your local antenatal or pregnancy clinic to enquire about models of care available in your area. You may also find midwives working in the community, so it is worth doing a Google search to see what is available. There are often posts on social media groups asking about midwives or doctors available in the area, so that could also be an avenue for finding a CoC model of care.

When you are looking for a CoC model, it is worth exploring a few key issues.

» Where do they offer appointments and how long are they?

» Do they work in a team? Who is their back up? Will you get to meet the other team members?

» Where do they offer birth services? What hospital/birth centre/ homebirth services are available?

» How will they *support you* to have a VBAC/repeat caesarean?

You may have specific questions that you want to add to this list, which is fine but is important you remain respectful towards the midwife or doctor. Always remember that a successful CoC relationship is a two-way relationship. The midwife or doctor needs to treat you with kindness and respect, but the same is also required; you need to treat them with kindness and respect too.

Choosing a Doula

It can be beneficial to also include a doula in your birth team. The role of the doula is varied and often individual to each doula, but they predominantly offer birth support to women and their families during labour and birth. Doula's have usually attended specific education and can become certified doulas. Doulas are not registered health professionals like midwives or doctors.

There is good research to support the use of a doula and having the support of a doula can reduce caesarean rates, decrease use of epidurals and pain relief, and decrease the length of labour and hospital stays (Adams & Curtin-Bowen, 2021; Bohren et al., 2017; Kozhimannil et al., 2016).

Research has looked at the impact of having a doula in a myriad of different situations, such as migrant women (Akhavan & Edge, 2012; Byrskog et al., 2020), low socioeconomic status (Darwin et al., 2017; Kozhimannil & Hardeman, 2016; McLeish & Redshaw, 2019), women of colour (Hardeman & Kozhimannil, 2016; Thomas et al., 2017), and women with intellectual disabilities (McGarry et al., 2016).

These studies show that having a doula can increase women's confidence in birthing and parenting, develop into trusting relationships, assist with making informed choices, and have positive impacts on emotional wellbeing.

Doulas can be hired privately, and the costs will vary on your area and what support you are looking for. There are some volunteer doula programs in some hospitals, so it is worth asking if this is offered near you.

You can find doulas in your area via Google, and there are also some "find a doula" websites. Below are some useful links regarding doulas.

» DONA International: https://www.dona.org/

» Doula Network Australia: https://www.doulanetwork.org/

» Doula UK: https://doula.org.uk/

Summary

This chapter has explored the importance of choosing the right maternity team to be by your side on your journey to a better birth. Different models of care have been explored and the benefits of continuity of care have been shown. In the next chapter, I will look at how important preparing for and having an active labour is for women planning a VBAC.

HAVING A GREAT TEAM CHECKLIST

- ☑ **Choose the team who are going to be on your side for your birth.**
- ☑ **Look for midwifery continuity of care models in your area.**
- ☑ **Consider hiring a doula.**

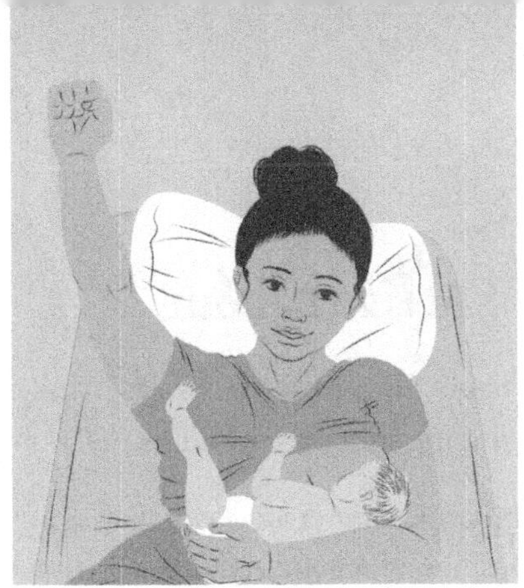

Chapter 8

HAVING AN ACTIVE LABOUR

When you think of a woman in labour and birthing, what do you see? Do you see a woman on a bed or standing? Is she squatting or does she have her legs in stirrups? What if you think back to pre-hospital times? What positions do you think of then?

Women traditionally used movement, rhythm, and upright birthing positions during labour and birth but this has more commonly been replaced with restricted movement, constant monitoring, and birthing on the bed. In Australia today, the most common birth position for women planning a VBAC is lying back in the bed (Keedle et al., 2020).

In this chapter, I will discuss the importance of being active in labour, how to prepare for being active in labour, and suggestions on how you can be active in labour, even with policy restrictions. This chapter has some amazing pictures drawn for this book by Ken Tackett. They are to inspire you to try out different positions and stay off the bed.

Importance of Active Labour

Researchers have been able to demonstrate the importance of being upright and active during labour and birth. A Cochrane Review found:

> *There is clear and important evidence that walking and upright positions in the first stage of labour reduces the duration of labour, the risk of caesarean birth, the need for epidural, and does not seem to be associated with increased intervention or negative effects on mothers' and babies' well-being* (Lawrence et al., 2013, p. 2).

The alternative to being active in labour is staying on the bed in semi-upright or lying-down positions. This is often paired up with having an epidural, which can increase the likelihood of assisted births, longer labours, more use of syntocinon/picoticin, and less breastfeeding rates (Newnham et al., 2020).

During phase two of my PhD, I found that women who had been active and upright during labour felt more resolved after the birth, regardless of whether that was vaginal or caesarean. Being active was seen as either contributing to having a VBAC or seen as trying all the options if a repeat caesarean was needed. The quote below describes this sentiment exactly.

> *I literally tried everything. I feel like if I ... so the whole time I was like, "oh, what if I did this in my first birth? What if I did that?" I tried everything I wanted to try that time this time and obviously there was no changing the outcome. So, I did what I could, and it still happened the same way. So obviously, there's nothing more I could have tried* (Angela, PN, Priv Obst) (Keedle et al., 2019, p. 10).

In the VBAC in Australia survey, we found the most common way to stay active in labour were position changes (75%), breathing techniques (58%), and using the shower (39%). The most common forms of pain relief were nitrous oxide (39%), epidural (20%), or not using any pain relief (25%). Women who had continuity of care with a midwife had higher rates of not using pain relief, upright birth, and waterbirth compared to continuity of care with a doctor or fragmented care (Keedle et al., 2020).

Preparation is the key to being active in labour and birth, and there are a variety of ways to get prepared.

Preparing for Being Active

In the VBAC in Australia survey, 52% of women stated that they accessed active labour resources. These varied from active labour classes to reading books. There is great variety in preparation for birth classes. Some classes are held in hospitals, clinics, birth centres, community centres, and especially since COVID-19, online. There is also great variety in the usefulness and effectiveness of these classes.

Traditional hospital classes can have more medical and pharmaceutical content (Levett & Dahlen, 2019), offering women a menu of drugs available and less information on natural methods of coping with labour and being active. This has led to non-hospital-based courses developed by childbirth educators, midwives, doulas, and complementary therapists that focused on active labour and birth, breathing techniques, and complementary therapies.

A randomised control trial from Sydney comparing hospital-based antenatal classes to classes teaching complementary therapies for women planning their first birth had interesting results (Levett et al., 2016b). The complementary-therapy classes included education on acupressure, visualisation and relaxation, breathing, massage, yoga, and facilitated partner support. Levett et al. (2016b) found the group that attended the complementary-therapy classes had decreased epidural, augmentation, caesarean, perineal trauma, and resuscitation of the baby rates alongside shorter length of second stage of labour. The women and partners that attended the course were interviewed and they highlighted how the information they gained provided them with a toolkit of techniques they could use when in labour, and that they had a deeper understanding about the physiological process of labour and birth (Levett et al., 2016a).

In response to this amazing work by Kate Levett, for her PhD, she is currently working with hospitals to introduce complementary-therapy classes into antenatal education programs. Although, all the women were expecting their first child and not planning a VBAC, this is significant research and supports the use of complementary-therapy-based labour and birth classes.

I do suggest you review the content of the course before paying any money. There are courses that suggest they can guarantee you the birth of your dreams just by following their advice, without giving you any actual tools and methods that you can use. There is also no method that can 100% guarantee you a vaginal birth so please be aware of that. Attending a reputable complementary- therapies education class that covers theory and different methods. It also covers techniques that you can use during labour can help you gain confidence in your ability to have a vaginal birth after caesarean and having a variety of different tools to use during your labour and birth.

There are a variety of organisations that offer complementary therapy-based labour and birth classes. Some examples and links are available in Table 3.

Table 3 – Country specific active labour class organisations

Country	Organization	Website
Australia	Calmbirth	https://calmbirth.com.au/
	Hypnobirthing Australia	https://hypnobirthingaustralia.com.au/
	She Births	https://shebirths.com/
USA	Lamaze	https://www.lamaze.org/
UK	National Childbirth Trust (NCT)	https://www.nct.org.uk/

How to Be Active in Labour When Monitored (CTG)

There are many different positions women can use to be upright and active. In this section, we will look at ways you can be active even with restrictions, such as a continuous fetal heart rate monitor or cardiotocography (CTG).

As identified in the section on uterine rupture in Chapter 3, continuous CTG monitoring is recommended practice in most hospital policies and guidelines. You can request not to have a CTG but that can be difficult to negotiate. For women planning to have a VBAC at home or in a birth centre, there is more likely going to be a handheld Doppler or Pinard fetoscope used for intermittent (auscultation) listening to the baby's heartbeat.

Having a CTG does not mean you can't be active. It is your right to be as active and upright as you want to be. There are a variety of CTGs available, and it is a good idea to ask your midwife or doctor what they have in their birthing unit. This can give you extra knowledge to help you prepare for being active in labour.

The traditional CTG is wired and has two transducers that are held on to the abdomen with elastic belts. One transducer measures the strength of contractions, and one measures the fetal heart rate. The meter length wiring can restrict movement but remember, the CTG machine is often on a wheeled trolley and has wiring, so it can be moved as well.

An excellent upright position, whether you have a wired CTG or not, is using the bed to lean on with you standing. Most hospital beds are electric, and you can raise it to be the best height for you to lean forward on. You can do this standing but also sitting on a birth ball. The two pictures below show how you can do this. These positions can also be a great way to ask your support person or midwife to put pressure or massage your lower back.

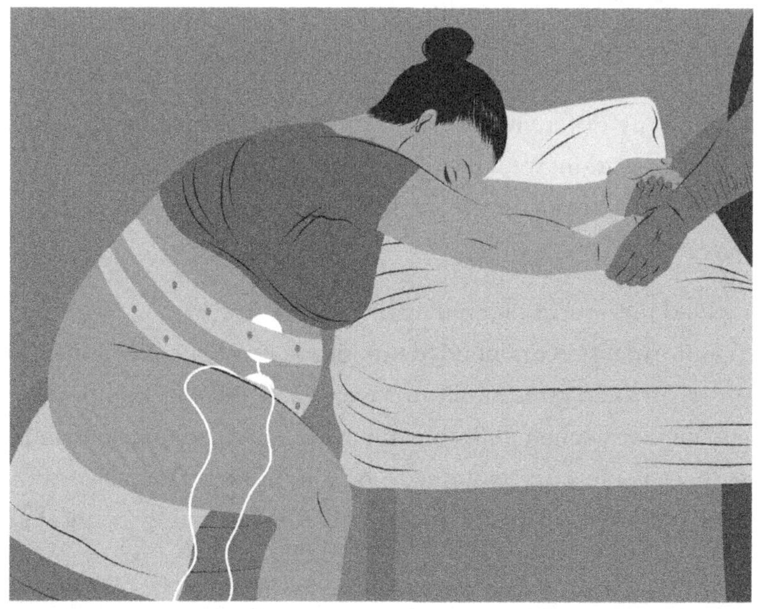

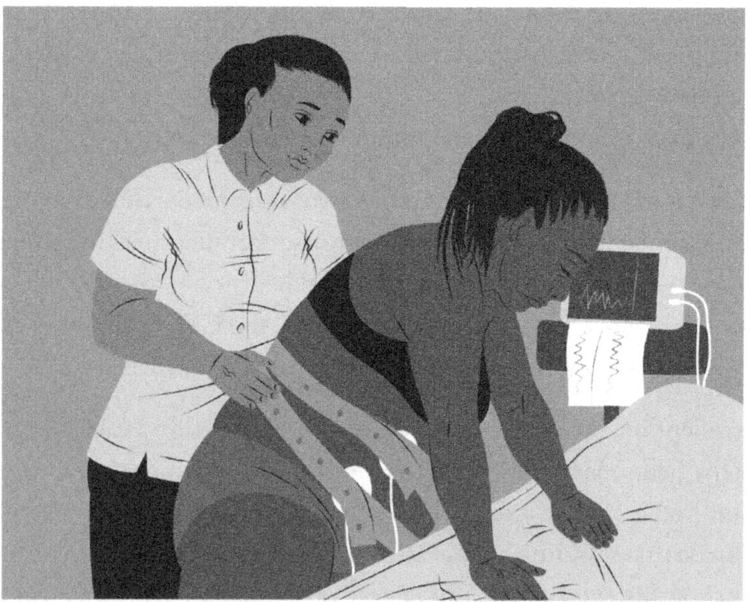

Some hospitals have access to wireless CTG machines. These CTG still have two transducers that are strapped round the abdomen but the data is transmitted wirelessly to the CTG machine (Watson et al., 2018).

A study of Australian midwives found that using a wireless CTG had positive impacts on women's sense of choice and control and freedom of movement in labour (Fox et al., 2020). There is research being undertaken using a new form of monitoring from Phillips that is wireless and beltless, called "non-invasive fetal electrocardiogram" (NIFECG) (Fox et al., 2021). Initial findings are promising and have found the NIFECG needs less fiddling with by midwives and enables greater freedom and movement by women. However, it isn't waterproof.

With a wireless CTG, you can walk around, use the birth mat on the floor, and use the shower. From my own experience as a midwife, I found that the water from the shower going directly onto the transducers could interfere with the trace but the water going down the back was fine for the trace and often preferred by women. The pictures below show a woman walking around with the support of her support person and being in the shower.

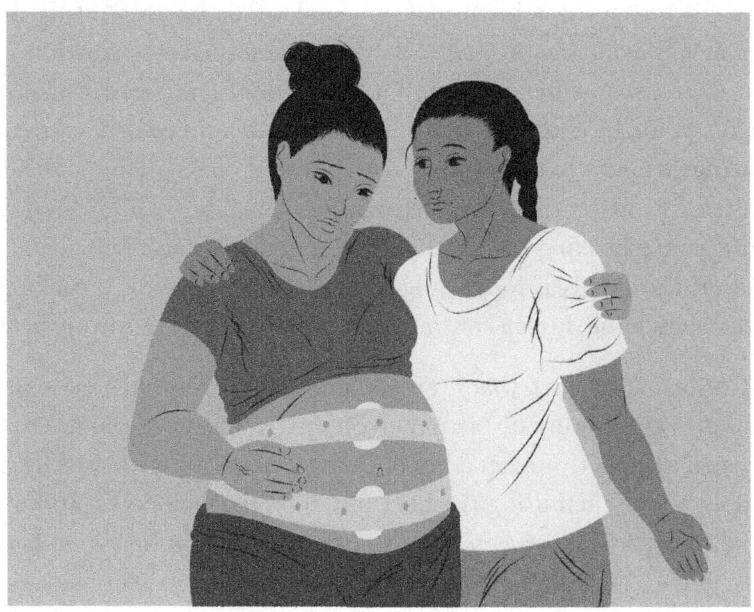

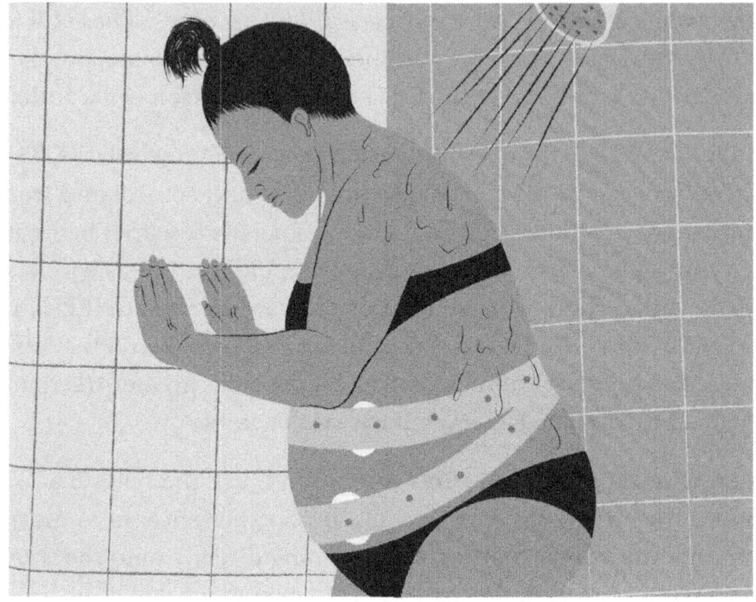

There will be the need during labour to get into rest positions and that doesn't need to be on the bed. A position I used a lot when I worked in hospitals was using a birth mat on the floor, or mattress of the bed if no mat was available. Actually, it was comfier and more cushioning for your knees, so go ahead and pull it off the bed. The partner or support person would be at the head of the woman, sometimes sitting on a chair or using cushions to sit on. The woman would be on all fours and could rest their head on their support person's lap. This would often result in the gentle stroking from the partner, which was also beneficial. This position can be great for resting in between contractions, rocking the hips, and moving during contractions. It is also a great birthing position.

A transformative birth that I remember fondly was when a woman who had a previous traumatic birth then birthed in this position. As the baby crowned, she gently lowered her bottom to the mat and birthed her baby without anyone handling the bub. She then reached down and picked up her baby from between her legs and sat down in disbelief. It was a truly magical experience for everyone in the room. The next picture gives an example of this position for labour.

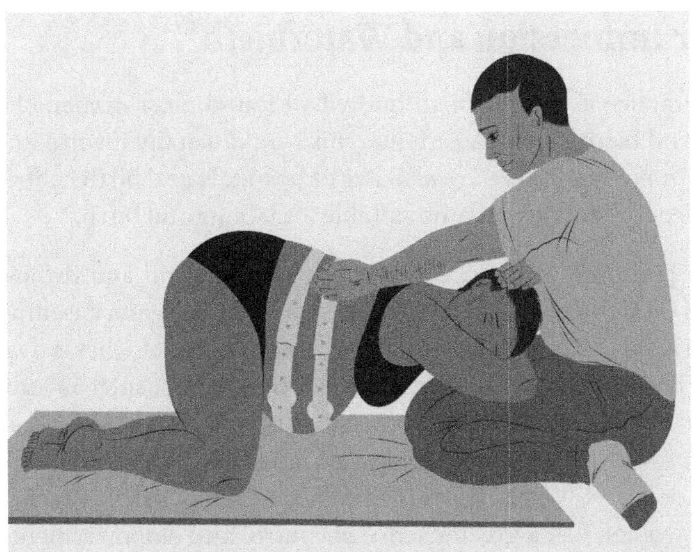

Other positions that keep you active and upright can include sitting on the toilet, sitting on a birthing stool, hanging onto rope, or anything that works for you. The picture below shows a woman on a toilet having intermittent auscultation with a Doppler.

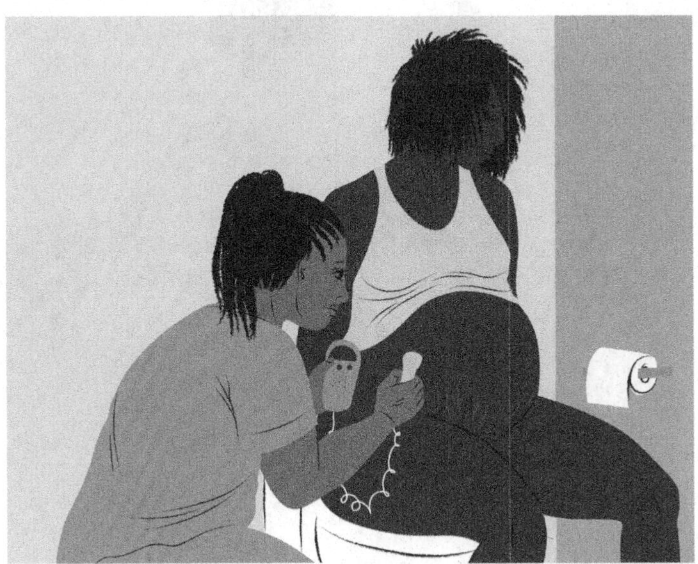

Water Immersion and Waterbirth

In my practice as a homebirth midwife, I found most women chose to labour and birth in water. At home this would usually involve an inflatable birth pool but there are also lots of hospitals and birth centres that have purpose built deep baths suitable for labour and birth.

Women planning a VBAC can use water immersion and in hospitals, wireless CTGs can be used, as they are waterproof. Again, it is important to discuss this with your midwife or doctor to find out what is available to you. There are many benefits to water immersion, such as improved freedom of movement and buoyancy, assisting with pain relief, soothing and improved relaxation, and shorter labours (Carlsson & Ulfsdottir, 2020; Cooper & Warland, 2019; Hodgson et al., 2020). Studies also suggest women feel a greater sense of control and empowerment when using water immersion (Clews et al., 2019; Fair et al., 2020). Studies have shown there is no greater risk of harm to babies born into water compared to not being born in water (Dahlen et al., 2013; Hodgson et al., 2020).

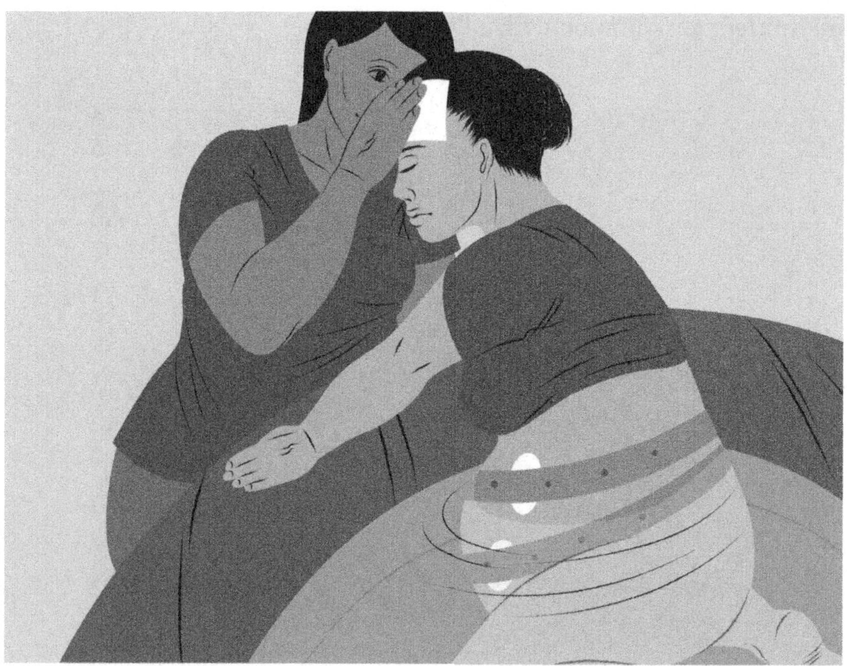

A study from Scotland reported on the experiences of women who used water immersion when planning a VBAC in a midwife-led unit (McKenna & Symon, 2014). Like the studies above, the women in this study reported improved feelings of support, comfort, mobility and relaxation, better pain relief, and a more positive attitude towards birth.

Wireless CTGs can be used in water and the previous image shows a woman in labour leaning forward onto the side of a birthing pool with a support person providing cold compresses to the forehead.

Summary

In this chapter, I have explored the importance of being active in labour, how to get knowledgeable about being active and using complementary therapies in labour, what positions you could do to promote active labour, and given information about the benefits of water immersion.

HAVING AN ACTIVE LABOUR CHECKLIST

- ☑ **Having an active labour checklist.**
- ☑ **Learn about how to be active in labour, consider going to classes.**
- ☑ **Be prepared to be active in labour, even with CTG, etc.**
- ☑ **Consider water immersion for labour and birth.**

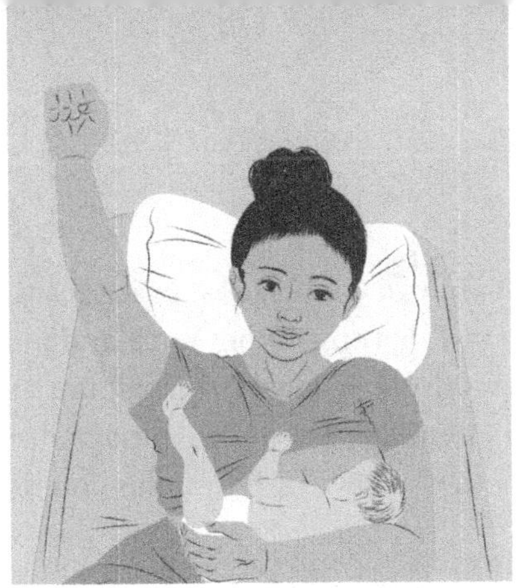

Chapter 9

PLANNING FOR A GENTLE CAESAREAN

You may decide that the best birth for you is to plan a repeat elective caesarean, or you may be thinking about what is important to you if you need a repeat emergency caesarean during labour. You can plan for a better caesarean experience and in this chapter, I will explore some decisions and factors you may find important to include.

What Does a Gentle Caesarean Look Like?

I use the term "gentle caesarean" as an umbrella term that encompasses whatever is important to you. In my research, when women reflected on their previous caesarean, they were often in bright and scary places with lots of unknown people and a sense of urgency and fear. They sounded far from gentle and a big shock after being in a quieter birthing room.

Most caesareans are not category 1, life-or-death, situations, and even if classified as an emergency, often take a little while to occur. An elective caesarean is different, as it is booked prior to labour occurring.

Even with a caesarean, you can request practices that will help you feel in more control of your birthing experience and make the event gentler. If you have done the three scenarios birth plan exercise in Chapter 5, you may be able to identify some of the important factors to you on the "worst-case-made-better" drawing. Examples could include:

» Lowering the lights

» Reduced unnecessary talking

» Playing your choice of music

» Having your support person of choice next to you

» Having a maternal assisted caesarean

» Asking for delayed cord clamping

» Having skin to skin in theatre

» Asking for a longer umbilical cord so you can use a cord tie of your choice

Maternal-Assisted Caesarean

A maternal-assisted caesarean (MAC) occurs when the screen is lowered, and the woman is assisted to reach down to the incision area (or close) and help pull out the baby from the uterus. The woman is then able to put the baby straight onto her chest.

Dr Jeni Stevens explored the experiences of women having skin to skin in theatre for her PhD and one of the women in her study was given the option to have a MAC. Jeni wrote about it in her PhD, but also in an article published in the now out-of-print magazine, *Midwifery Matters*.

In this article, Jeni describes the process the woman went through to have her MAC, such as doing a surgical scrub of her hands and putting on sterile gloves, the placements of monitoring equipment on areas of her body that wouldn't be restrictive to holding her baby, the drape lowered for the woman to reach down and then lifted once she had put the baby on her chest, and the midwife drying and cutting the cord with the baby on the woman's chest (Stevens, 2015). This MAC was the first one performed at the hospital and Jeni writes about how joyful and emotional the event was for the woman and her partner. The woman was able to hold her baby for over 2 hours without separation and breast fed within 5 minutes. The facilitator of this MAC was the obstetrician, and they were key to ensuring it went ahead. In Jeni's PhD thesis there is a quote from the woman about her MAC.

> *That was really, really exciting to have him and deliver him the way that I did. Within the first, I think it was 5 minutes or so, I was breast-feeding, got an opportunity to have that one-on-one contact. I just couldn't stop looking at him. I was in disbelief a lot of the time. For that experience, I'd treasure forever* (Stevens, 2018, p. 107).

There is a lack of research on MAC and the availability varies amongst obstetricians and hospitals. There is also a lot of mixed feelings about this practice from women and healthcare providers, but ultimately, if you feel this would help you feel more in control and confident in your birth choices, then you should talk with your midwife and/or doctor about this option.

Skin to Skin in Theatre

Skin to skin in theatre is where the baby is placed onto the woman's chest, the baby is naked, and the woman's chest is bare. Studies on skin to skin in theatre have shown that the stress levels of women decrease and comfort and oxytocin levels increase when having skin to skin, with no negative outcomes for babies (Frederick et al., 2020).

Your hospital may or may not offer skin to skin in theatre, as there are a variety of practices from hospital to hospital. Although research identifies how important and wanted skin to skin in theatre is for women and their partners (Stevens et al., 2019), barriers can include a lack of support and a lack of education on the benefits of skin to skin in theatre from healthcare professionals in theatre, such as midwives and nurses (Stevens et al., 2018).

It is important to talk to your midwife or doctor during your pregnancy about your wishes for skin to skin in theatre and emphasis how important it is for you. Find out if this will be available to you and question why if it is not. If they say no and you have the resources, then speak to managers in that hospital or other healthcare providers and hospitals to see if another one local to you does provide this service. Sometimes, it takes the first one to occur to be the facilitator for skin to skin in theatre to become an available practice for other women.

Summary

You can plan for a better caesarean experience if you choose or need to have a caesarean. Consider what made the caesarean difficult for you before and then what is important for you this time to help you feel more in control and confident about your birthing experience. Planning for a gentle caesarean can be different for each person but ensure you talk to your midwife or doctor during your pregnancy about your plans and wishes so these can be taken into consideration and implemented in time for your birthing experience.

HAVING A GENTLE CAESAREAN CHECKLIST

- ☑ **Think about what a gentle caesarean means for you.**
- ☑ **Talk to your healthcare provider about your gentle caesarean wishes.**
- ☑ **Remind your healthcare provider on the day about your wishes.**

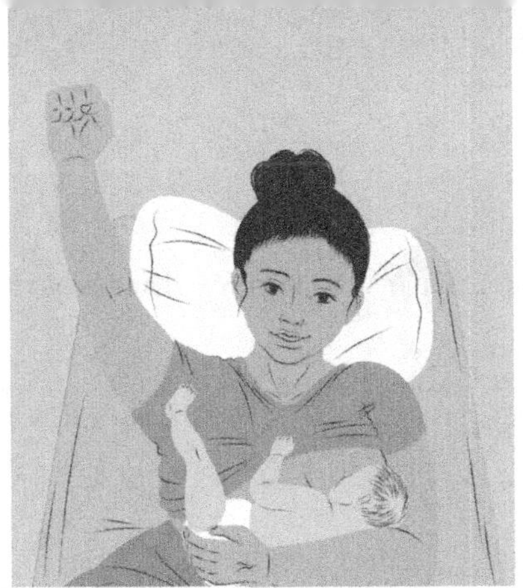

Chapter 10

WOMEN'S STORIES

In this chapter, I share with you women's stories of having a birth after a caesarean. I put a post on my social media page and within days, I had many stories to share with you. I am grateful to the women that shared their stories and I hope they give you inspiration and motivation to plan for the best birth for you.

i stand in front of the mirror, and run my fingers across the scar.
three years later,
and it is still sensitive to touch.
i used to hate this scar.
and all it represented.
my body failing.
how you entered this world.
i hated it all.
but now, it's magic.
a magical portal that brought you to me.
it is strength.
as i lay down on a cold operating table,
bright lights.
as they cut me open,
shaking and shivering.
i did it.
i'll do it again.
anything to have you in my arms.
this scar is magic.
it is a sign that you were
once part of me.
that you came from me.
i love this scar.
it is magic
like you.

emineh

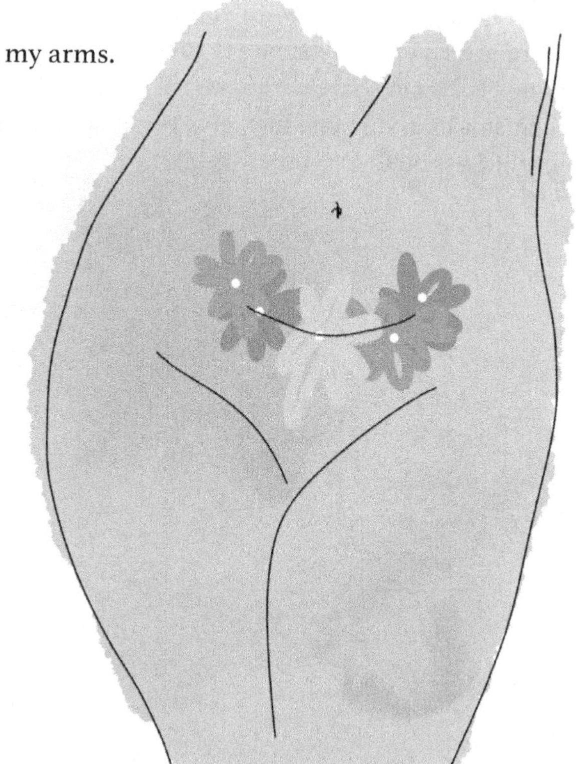

your birth was different.
so different to my first.
it was calm. it was peaceful.
i was in control.
it was beautiful.
it was healing.
i felt as if i crossed into the heavens,
and brought you home,
into my arms.
i felt angels around me.
i felt the power of prayer.
i felt strong.
your birth healed me,
my sweet boy.
thank you.

emineh

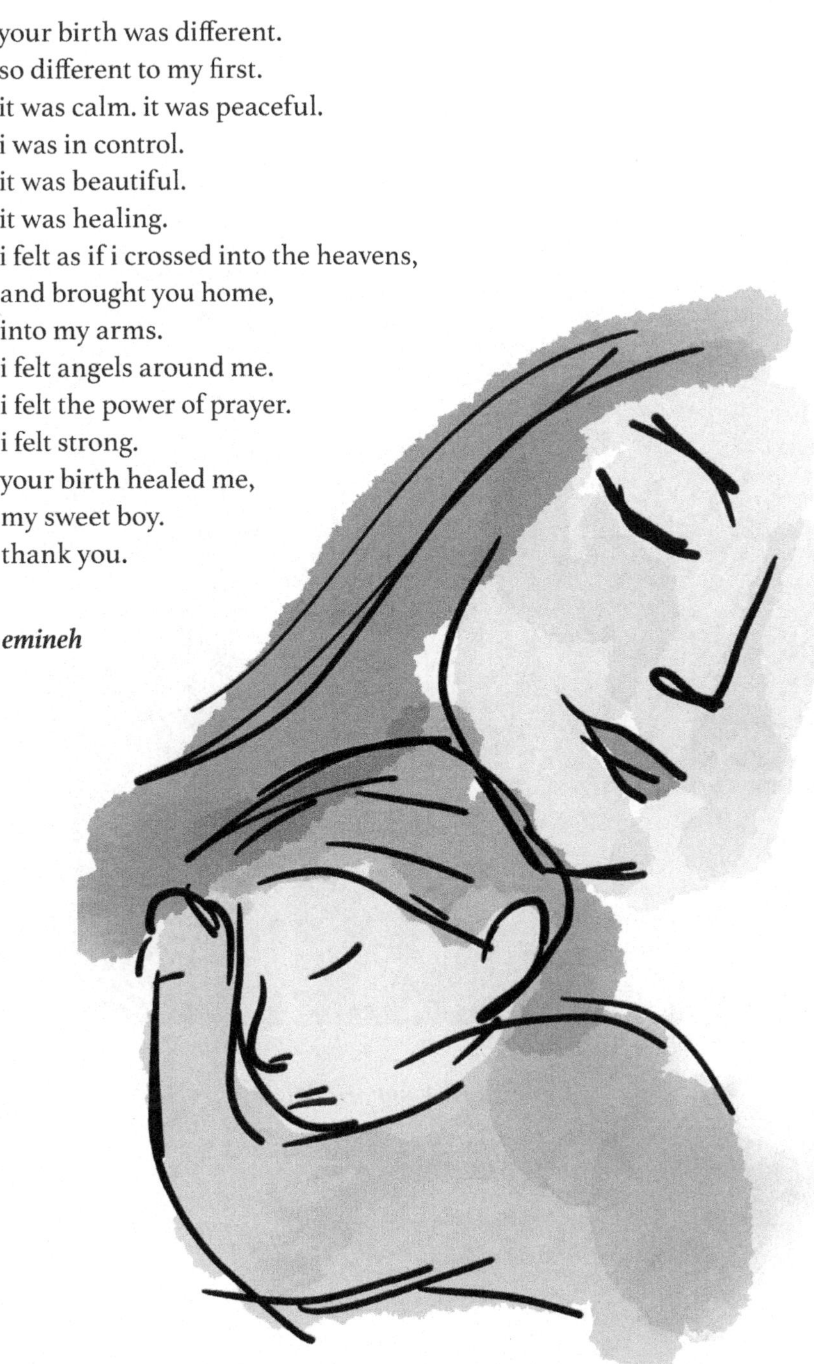

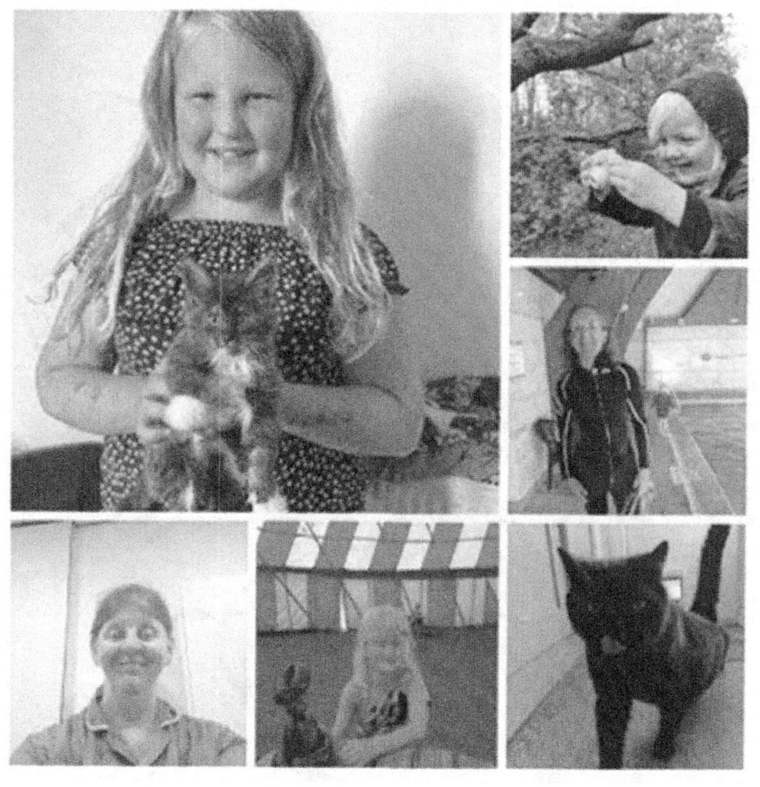

Caroline Hickman, Hull, UK

Caroline - VBAC with a Classical Scar

I have 3 beautiful children; 1 girl, Sophie, aged 9, and 2 boys, Thomas and Noah, aged 6 and 2. My pregnancy with Sophie was textbook and I gave birth at 40+2, and Sophie was born on Father's Day on June 19th, 2011. I was induced after my waters broke on June 18th and nothing happened. 10 hours later, Sophie arrived after induction and a forceps delivery. I had a tiny bit of gas and air at the end but used hypnobirthing, mainly. After Sophie, I got the baby blues.

My pregnancy with Thomas was fine until I had my bloods done for Down syndrome, as I was older, at 38. It came back as high risk at a 1:14 chance of a Down syndrome baby. I had the amniocentesis done, as I was old, and it was negative. Everything else was fine until I was 28 weeks, and my waters broke at 6 am. I was sleepy and thought I had wet myself initially, and went back to bed, moving over to Mark's side. 10 minutes later, his side of the bed was wet. I went through to the bathroom, where Mark was getting ready for an early shift, and there, my waters went good and proper. We called the labour ward and they said to go in straight away. There, I stayed until Friday. It was Sunday when it all kicked off. I was admitted and monitored. I went up and down between the ante-natal ward and the labour ward for 24 hours, until I went into labour. I was re-admitted to the labour ward and the midwife who was looking after me was horrible. She didn't introduce herself, and to this day I don't know her name. I was examined by the doctor, and she told me my baby was transverse and I needed a category-1 emergency c-section. I was rushed to theatre and given a spinal, and Thomas was born at 6:02 pm by classical c-section, weighing 2lbs, 6oz. Mark got to hold him briefly. My first glimpse of him was as he was taken to the NICU. I didn't see him until 2 the following morning. I had to wait until I could get into a wheelchair and the spinal had worn off.

I was able to hold him 5 days later, for the first time, in high dependency. He had spent the first 5 days in intensive care. He spent 25 days in high dependency and 50 days in special care. 80 looooong days. During those 80 days, I fell apart physically and mentally. I picked up a urine, wound, and bowel infection. I ended up back in hospital briefly when my wound opened up and got no sympathy from the midwives. I had to go back to the postnatal ward for my wound checks. I waited ages and got forgotten about several times. Not one of the midwives who saw me asked me how I was doing.

I was falling apart, mentally. 3 weeks after Thomas was born, I ended up at the GP surgery, having dark thoughts about jumping off the Humber Bridge. I ended up being referred to the perinatal mental health team and was put on antidepressants. The health visitor did a new baby visit and asked me where the baby was. She and the student health visitor gasped in shock when I told them where he was. No one had communicated that to them. They should have done their sums, because I had been to see a different one the week before to get my red book at 27 weeks.

The perinatal team were a mixed blessing. I suffered with severe postnatal depression, and it was awful. I struggled to bond with Thomas until he got into special care, as I was scared that he would die. Why on earth would I bond with a baby that might die? The only thing that kept me going was the thought that I needed to stay alive to breastfeed the baby—he had done nothing wrong and deserved my milk—and I was the only one who could do it. So, I expressed and expressed until I was able to feed him. I was so fed up with that bloody pump and ready to throw it out of the window. To make matters worse, NICU was opposite the dialysis unit, where I worked at the time.

The trust made me start my maternity leave the day after Thomas was born because I gave birth after 28 weeks. 28 weeks and 1 day. If I had given birth at 27 week and 6 days, I could have spilt my maternity leave. But no, the trust stuck to their policy and that was that. It was policy, end of. This caused me a lot of grief, as it wasn't maternity leave but a living hell. I felt normal for the first time, when I was able to feed Thomas myself. Breastfeeding is so important for those happy hormones. There was no way on this earth that my baby—I had bonded by this time—was going to have any crappy formula. I continued to feed Thomas until he was 15 months old.

NICU, in their wisdom, referred me to social services as *support.* They were completely awful and gave us, as family, a hard time, and couldn't understand, and had no compassion or empathy. They were evil. Eventually we got rid of them. They were hung up about Thomas' weight and wanted me to bottle feed. They threatened me with Thomas' brain not developing. Total crap! Today, he is as bright as a button.

I went to see the consultant who delivered Sophie and was there when I was on the antenatal ward. He told me that no obstetrician would let me deliver naturally again and I would *have* to have a planned c-section. I thought, "on your bike, mate."

Even after all this, I still desperately wanted another baby, so I read a book about an independent midwife and began searching and found Yorkshire Storks. It was important to me to have complete continuity of care after my experiences with Thomas. I wanted to get to know the midwives and them get to know me. I wanted to avoid the hospital as much as I could, as it gave me terrible anxiety, especially near the NICU. I had shared care with the Storks and the NHS. The NHS gave me so much grief about me wanting a home birth, as I was so high risk due to my classical c-section. I ended up having to go for an appointment with 2 consultants, who were awful, especially the male consultant. He was arrogant. If I agreed to a hospital birth, it would be the labour ward only and I wouldn't be able to have a water birth. It would be monitored and totally medical, which was everything I wanted to avoid.

I was able to have all my Storks appointments in my own home – so much more relaxing and stress free. I got to know them all well. They felt like a little family to me. Sophie and Thomas could be there, and Frankie the cat too. I had no restrictions at all or any hospital policy to conform to. They gave me information about the special scars Facebook group, and I got lots of information and support from them. I was able to chat to lots of other mums who had done what I was planning to do and totally understood all the scare tactics the medics were giving me about how I could die, and I was being reckless. They gave me the percentages about the risk of uterine rupture up to 10%, depending on what research you read. Well, turn that on its head and it's a 90% chance of it *not* happening. Add to that the cascade of intervention that the hospital staff have to be seen to be doing something all the time. It was something I wasn't comfortable with. I wanted a gentle home birth with my children around me, and Frankie. I wanted to be in my own environment, as it's much more relaxing. I wanted oxytocin to do its thing, *not* the stress hormone adrenaline.

When I eventually did go into labour at 41+4 at 11:45pm on November 9th, I knew I didn't have to worry about whether the home birth team would have enough staff to send anyone out to me or whether I had met them or not before. I could choose who to ring from the team of 4 Storks, I would know them, and they would be available. I rang Sharyn, as I had seen her earlier that day. She contacted Chris and they headed over. My husband Mark had been up to Scotland for a job interview that day and had got home at 8pm, having got up at 4am and left at 5am. He was shattered, bless him. We had nicknamed our bump Herbert and I had said to Herbert, "please, wait until Daddy gets home before you choose to come." Well, he did wait but only just. Poor Mark. We put Sophie and Thomas to bed and had a bath, and I said to Mark, "for your sake, I hope Herbert doesn't come tonight." We got into bed, and I was snoring and sleeping on my left-hand side, and keeping Mark awake, so I turned over and at that point, my waters broke.

Mark got out of bed, I ran the bath and rang Sharyn, and Mark started getting the pool ready. He attached my TENS machine to my back, and I started using it straight away. This was from about 12 am to 3am; we used the hypno-birthing scripts, had low lighting, and gentle baby lullabies playing. Mark had a soothing voice, as he was doing the hypnobirthing. He admits now he was winging it. I just needed his voice. Sophie, Noah, and Thomas love his storytelling voice now. We were alone, just the 2 of us, and it was quite surreal – so different to the other births I had had, and then, Chris arrived first, followed shortly by Sharyn. I was in the pool by the time they arrived. They started knitting and chilling out, and I continued my breathing and relaxation. They were there but not there, if that makes sense. I felt completely calm if they were knitting. Everything must be alright then, and I didn't need to worry if they weren't.

About 4:30am, we woke Sophie up. I had asked both of them if they wanted waking up if Herbert came in the middle of the night. Sophie said, "definitely" and Thomas said, "absolutely not." Sophie watched me give birth and she told me that we had a baby boy, and his name was Noah Francis. Noah was born at 5:02am and weighed 10.1lbs. I had no stitches or tearing. Sophie went back to bed at this point. I delivered the placenta naturally and then laid on the sofa and had tea and toast. It was delicious. Noah had his first few suckles, and I just lay, enjoying holding him. Around 7 am, Thomas came trotting down the stairs and said, "oh, Mummy, Herbert's here." It was just so beautiful to hear that from him and so natural.

Claire came later that day, and everything was just fab. I was in bed starting my babymoon, which I thoroughly enjoyed. It felt satisfying to know I had done it and proved the NHS consultants wrong with their threats and scaremongering. I just knew my body could do it, after all, I didn't need any help to get pregnant, so why should I need help to deliver my baby?

I didn't get even get the baby blues, let alone postnatal depression. I recovered quickly physically and there weren't any infections. My gut instinct told me everything was going to be fine, and it was. I fed Noah until he was 22 months. The postnatal care was amazing from the Storks and lasted until about 8 weeks. A far cry from what I experienced with Sophie and less so with Thomas. I got 3 visits with Sophie and no visits with Thomas.

We are now working on making our fourth and final baby and wouldn't hesitate to use independent midwives again. I will bypass the NHS altogether this time.

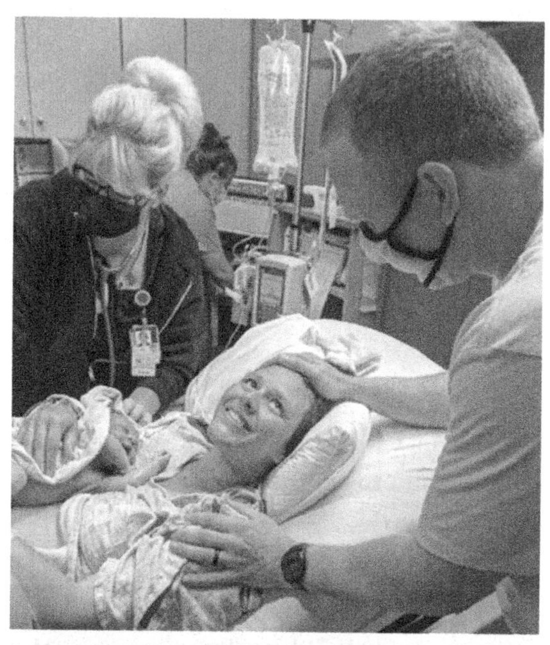

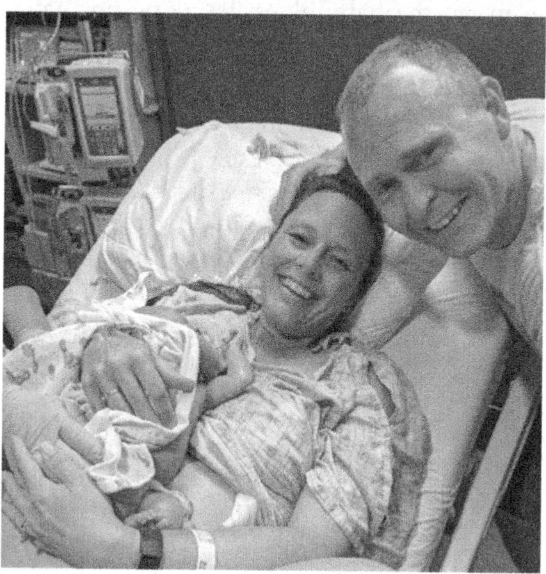

Kari Lammer, Iowa, USA

Kari – VBAC after a Uterine Rupture

My vaginal birth after my uterine rupture (VBAR) baby arrived on Monday, June 14, 2021. From our first c-section birth (2014) to our rupture baby (2017), to the decision to have another (2020), to finalizing a birth plan (2021), this has been a long journey for my husband and me. In the end, I wouldn't trade or change a single thing about this pregnancy and delivery.

It's hard to come up with the words to describe this birth. All I can say is that I expected this birth to go well. What I didn't expect was perfection.

Birth History

Our first baby was born via c-section. I was in early labor for about 8 to 9 hours before the clinic wanted me to come in and do a non-stress test (NST). The NST had some non-reassuring heart tones. They did a biophysical profile (BPP) and saw I had low fluid. The clinic sent me to the hospital, saying the doctor on call would discuss next steps and delivery options.

I was naive and trusting of whatever the doctor said. After being there for about two hours, the on-call doctor came in, saying he recommended a c-section because our baby was at risk of brain damage or death. At the time, it was an easy decision.

I remember being so scared and alone in the operating room. There was a wonderful nurse by my side, but it wasn't enough to remove the trauma from that c-section. Once the baby was born, he was admitted to the NICU for a pneumothorax (collection of air or gas in the space inside the chest around the lungs). I couldn't see him for 12 hours after delivery. Immediately after him being born, I was so thankful he was here, without brain damage and a now-healthy lung. I remember thanking the doctors for recognizing this risky situation and getting him out. But I also remember feeling cheated out of an experience, having no part in how he was born or delivered.

It wasn't until I was home and doing late-night nursing sessions that I was researching NSTs, BPPs, oligohydramnios, and everything about his birth, that I discovered c-sections are all too common and too often used for the convenience of doctors. I started to question how much of an emergency we were truly facing with our baby and birth. I should have been more informed. I should have asked more questions. Why did I blindly trust the recommendation?

After doing my research for our second baby, I was determined to have a vaginal birth after c-section (VBAC). I switched my care to a clinic with midwives. I read so many birth books, hired a doula, learned about natural birth, becoming a self-advocate, and learned how to navigate a hospital maternity system I had lost trust in. I decided on a Bradley birth and was prepared for a natural, hospital-based birth, trying to avoid any cascade of interventions.

This was an uneventful pregnancy, but I did have small low-grade fevers up until about 20 weeks. I'd have waves of light nausea that came with a small fever. Never enough to disrupt my daily life. Just a small inconvenience. I stayed active the entire pregnancy.

Then, in the third trimester, I was diagnosed with gestational diabetes. I was convinced the test was wrong. I ate an extremely low-carb diet at the time and was sure my body didn't know how to process the glucose, given that it was outside my normal diet. I decided not to modify my diet and just track my blood glucose. Luckily, every number was fine until week 39, when I had a few high post-meal numbers. Regardless of how well-controlled it was, it didn't change my midwife's recommendation to induce me at 39 weeks. Thank God I was more educated and said no. At 40 weeks, she wanted to induce me again. I said no but decided to start my maternity leave so I could mentally disconnect from work and focus on having a baby.

Early labor began the next morning, around 10 am. 4:30 pm-ish, active labor began. We went to the hospital at 6:30 pm. I got super relaxed in bed and basically slept until transition. Pushing started at 9 pm-ish. About 50 minutes into pushing, the baby crowned, then receded, and lost good heart tones. The doctor was called in with the midwife. I remember the midwife saying, "you need to push the baby out on this next contraction." The doctor had the vacuum ready and with the help of it, the baby was out on the next contraction. Her Apgar score was a two and she needed to be resuscitated with a CPAP machine.

Immediately after labor, I had trouble taking deep breaths, had pain in my right shoulder, felt like I had to hold my c-section scar when I was up walking around, and felt like there was something inside me that didn't belong. My stomach was distended and continued to get worse. I also didn't have any bowel movements and never started producing milk. They did two ultrasounds, looking for a rupture, but none was detected. Throughout all this, my vital signs never changed, and my hemoglobin stayed stable at 12 something. Although there were enough symptoms to have the medical team looking for a rupture, there just wasn't enough evidence for them to be confident it was a rupture. Therefore, I was discharged.

With my baby in the NICU, I was still rooming at the hospital. There were two nurses who saw my condition worsen (stomach getting more distended, losing color in my skin, having severe back pain) and, although I wasn't a patient, they tried to reach my midwife and the doctor on call. Before they heard back from either, they suggested I go to the ER. I wouldn't have gone on my own. If me and the baby were both at home, I would have waited and waited. But that day, when the nurse said she'd take me to the ER, I said yes. As I have reflected on that time, I believe those nurses saved my life.

We got right in at the ER. A scan showed my abdomen was full of fluid and I had developed an ileus (which explains the lack of a bowel movement). Next was an exploratory laparotomy to determine the most appropriate action.

Prayers from family and friends kicked into action right away as I was wheeled to surgery.

I remember asking the doctors to save my uterus, if possible, and praying that God's will be done, but also praying I'd wake up okay to be with Luke and my kids.

Sure enough, the laparotomy showed my c-section scar fully opened and I had 1600 cubic centimeters of blood and amniotic fluid in my abdomen (no need for a blood transfusion). Luckily, my rupture was contained to the previous scar, not extending anywhere else in my uterus.

A roller coaster of emotions followed. Going from one of the most empowering days of my life to one of the scariest was a lot to process.

That experience was much more traumatic for Luke than our first birth. For me, it was an ideal birth minus the rupture (despite the rupture, I had an amazing birth high). As to why the first c-section was more traumatic than the vaginal birth with a rupture, I don't know. I wonder if it has to do with the lack of control or a feeling of being taken advantage of (my fault for not being educated going into our first birth) from that c-section. Maybe it's simply the memory of being alone, the all-white-sterile room, not being able to see my baby. I'm just not sure.

We were undecided on a third going into our second birth, but with the rupture, there was even more to question if we were to have another. A hysterectomy was not needed. I was told I could have more children but would need to be delivered between 37 to 38 weeks via scheduled c-section.

Regardless, I knew if we had a third, I wanted another VBAC/VBAR. I joined the Special Scars Facebook group and learned of many people who go on to have vaginal births after doctors told them it wasn't possible based on their birth history. When I shared my story, I learned of a clinic that supported VBARS. I learned a ton more than that, but knowing it was possible gave me hope.

I did all sorts of things to prepare for a third baby, should we make that decision. I started seeing a therapist who specializes in birthing trauma. I started collagen and vitamin C supplements to strengthen my uterus. I read every piece of literature or study on pregnancy after rupture and ruptures in general. I joined a Facebook group that is for people who are interested in a vaginal birth post-rupture. It's not just me who wants this.

Although I immediately knew if we had a third that I would want a VBAR, below is what I learned about myself, ruptures, and risks:

I believe every pregnancy is different and just because a rupture happened once, that isn't a guarantee it will happen again. (I see plenty of birth stories from rupture moms who do a c-section, and her doctor says her uterus looks great. Then, there're moms who VBAC repeatedly and then rupture. There is never any guarantee.)

There is enough research to indicate a pregnancy was safe for my type of rupture and I was confident in my own health.

There are virtually no studies or research on vaginal births after ruptures. To me, if it hasn't been studied, how do we know it's not safe?

We know there are risks with a planned c-section at 37 to 38 weeks (both for Mom and baby).

Even if a rupture were to happen again, it doesn't mean it would be catastrophic. I was willing to do extra monitoring.

More important than what the research said, I wanted a say in how I'd deliver a future baby. It's my health and my baby. Luke and I should have a say in when and how a future baby is delivered. If I could repeat my births, I'd take my rupture birth over my c-section (maybe it goes back to the feeling of being in control). Knowing that uterine surgery was what led to my rupture, I'd do anything to avoid an elective c-section. I think most of all, I've learned to greatly trust my intuition and my intuition said, "go for it." That was not easy to explain to Luke, my doctors, or pretty much anyone.

I talked to my OB about a trial of labor and the reasons stated above. Speaking of my OB, he was the doctor who assisted the midwife when I delivered my rupture baby. He also happened to be at the hospital (not on call) when I went to the ER, and he decided to join the on-call doctor for my rupture surgery. So, he truly saw it all: my birth, my rupture, and my surgery. I honestly think he was entertaining the idea of a VBAR, but he referred me to a maternal-fetal medicine (MFM) specialist for an opinion. What was most notable was that he did not say no. He set us on the next leg of our journey of meeting with MFM.

The first MFM I saw didn't give any consideration to the research I had done, what I wanted from a future birth, how I felt, or what mattered to me. I was immediately dismissed. The short answer: why would you want this? You'll kill your baby and kill yourself. Honestly, there wasn't much of a long answer. Luke and I sat in a small exam room while three doctors stood over us, lecturing us on why this should be dismissed. I barely made it out of the clinic without bursting into tears. That was an absolutely terrible appointment, and I won't forget how I was treated and felt. That car ride home was hard.

Luckily, there was another MFM doctor I could see, so I got a second referral. This MFM restored my trust in the profession and words can't express how thankful I am for his support. He knew I did my research, understood the risks, and realized that how I felt mattered. He didn't think it was unreasonable to consider a VBAR.

The most important thing for me heading into a potential third birth was (while a vaginal birth was important to me, I needed the following):

Finding my voice.

Having a say in how I would deliver a baby.

Being a part of the decision-making process.

I wasn't opposed to a c-section if it was medically indicated, but until that time, I wanted a chance at labor. I wanted a team approach to birth, one that I, as the birthing patient, was a part of and didn't have to fight to have a voice or choice. My MFM was a critical part of the team.

Luke and I had two preconception visits with our new MFM. He said he'd support me and a trial of labor if we did, indeed, conceive. He said he'd pick out an OB who he thought would be supportive of the plan. He wanted me to deliver at a higher-level hospital than the one in my hometown and wanted to monitor the scar via ultrasound.

Luke and I started couples counseling to work through the trauma of our previous births and talk about future births while focusing on our relationship. Together, we arrived at the decision to try for another baby and agreed we wouldn't make any decisions about delivery too far in advance. We'd wait and see if our MFM found a supportive OB; we'd wait and see how the pregnancy developed; we'd wait and be part of the discussion with our doctor team. One step at a time.

Pregnancy After Rupture

We conceived in September 2020. I saw my general practitioner to confirm the pregnancy and scheduled a 12-week appointment with my MFM.

My first trimester was good. I had some nausea from about week 7 to week 12, but it was manageable. I was able to keep up my running routine as normal. In fact, on my birthday (11 weeks), I got a 9-mile run in.

When the time came for my 12-week appointment, my MFM measured my scar, which was 7mm*, and checked all the other normal pregnancy stuff. He then talked to an OB about taking on my care. She said "yes!" I couldn't believe it when I got the phone call. I had a supportive team, was being treated respectfully, was being listened to, and was part of my care!

*Regarding scar thickness, the literature my MFM and OB were referencing was a meta-analysis of several studies monitoring correlation of scar thickness in single, low-transverse c-sections, and risk of rupture.

At 14 weeks, I joined the Brewer Diet Facebook group and started to modify my diet to focus on high protein, initially aiming for 85 to 115 grams of protein per day and getting all the food groups in. The Brewer Diet taught me to eat a more balanced diet than I ever have before. With my rupture baby and eating style when not pregnant, I typically tried to avoid grains (rice, quinoa, whole wheat bread), little fats (butter, oil), any milk or cheese, trying to stick with a Weight Watchers diet of low or zero-point foods (and let's be real, saving all my points for chocolate on occasion). On the Brewer Diet, I adjusted to buttering my whole wheat egg sandwich, adding some rice or quinoa to my meals, and eating yogurt and cheese regularly (and more, but these are just notable examples for me).

After the first trimester, I added in Maya Abdominal Self-Care massage (I saw a professional with my second but didn't do the full treatment with this one because of COVID).

The second trimester was not notable, in a good way. I started my formal Bradley classes (I loved my first Bradley birth and wanted to take the class, which wasn't available in my area at the time of my previous birth) and started my birth book reading. I had a 20-week ultrasound with MFM where my scar was measured. I will say that I was surprised about how much it thinned from 12 weeks to 20 weeks, which was 3 mm.

However, I wasn't worried yet. I knew my MFM comfort level was 2 mm and although, he had previously stated his recommendation, he continually reassured me that everything would be okay. I also had no idea what to expect in terms of the rate of thinning throughout the pregnancy. So, I just accepted the 3 mm and continued on my path. Still extremely focused on Brewer Diet (I allowed myself one cheat day per month), hitting my protein goals, continuing running, massaging my scar, doing pregnancy stretches/exercises, and taking collagen and vitamin C supplements.

At my 24-week appointment, my OB had reviewed the 20-week ultrasound and shared a little discomfort with the 3 mm. Where my MFM was comfortable with a trial of labor at 2 mm, she was more comfortable with 3 mm, which is where I was at already. She also said that maybe that measurement was with a full bladder, so that made me think my OB and MFM were going to measure in different ways. She said she'd do her own ultrasound at 30 and 36 weeks to see what she thinks.

A lot of this gave me anxiety; the thought of a new person and new equipment doing measurements at 30 and 36 weeks. Were my OB and MFM measuring the same way? What's the comfort level of the team in proceeding with the labor plan? I called my MFM clinic in a slight panic, but the nurse calmed me down, helped me understand how insurance would work and that I could keep my 28-week appointment with their clinic. I'd be lying if I didn't start questioning if my plan was going to work or start thinking about "what-ifs."

My 28-week appointment was another ultrasound with my MFM. I saw the nurse who I'd talked to a few weeks earlier. She made a point to check on my wellbeing, reading between the lines, and knowing I had some anxiety. She was just what I needed at that appointment.

I talked to my MFM about my OBs comfort level, her comment about my bladder being full, and concerns about switching to her ultrasounds after I've been through so much with him and his practice. We decided to continue with his measurements so I could have some consistency. We measured with an empty and full bladder, so however she measured, we'd have a comparison. He also wasn't surprised that she was more comfortable with 3 mm. He said he's looking at this from a research standpoint, where she is looking at it from a practical standpoint. At this appointment, my scar measured 2.5 mm with a full bladder and 5 mm on an empty bladder. They also noted mildly increased amniotic fluid. This had me a bit worried for my upcoming gestational diabetes test, but (I believe) thanks to the Brewer Diet and my well-balanced eating, I passed that with flying colors.

Following this appointment, I had a tour with the nurse manager of the hospital we'd be delivering at. I had a whole list of questions about how doctors and anesthesia handle call schedules, my options for a natural labor given I'd be showing up earlier than I would otherwise, COVID restrictions in place, time to the OR in the case of an emergency, a family centered c-section if needed, etc. That visit gave me so much confidence in our hospital choice. We were clearly in great hands.

After my 28-week appointment, I decided I needed to do more to ensure the delivery plan stayed on course. I couldn't just sit back and watch my opportunity slip away with my scar measuring 2.5 mm. This is also when Luke got more serious about the meta-analysis, understanding the terminology, thinking about my birth history, etc.

I added red raspberry leaf tea to my daily routine and picked up bone broth to start drinking. Between Luke and me, we were looking for the best ways to strengthen that tissue. As a weightlifter, he knew a lot about nutrition for muscle growth and as a passionate birthing person, I learned a fair amount about strengthening and toning the uterus.

My 30-week appointment was an ultrasound with my OB. She ended up measuring with a full bladder, transvaginally, where my MFM was measuring transabdominally. The scar measurement was 2.7 to 3.7 mm. It could be the difference in how they measured, but I was reassured by this measurement, given the small additions of tea and bone broth (for those two weeks, it was 1 cup of tea daily and sporadic bone broth drinking).

After this appointment, I was out on a run, which is when I do most of my thinking and self-reflection. I texted my husband:

> *I am going to do everything I can to get above 3 mm, going for 3.5. I'm going to stay doing 1 cup of bone broth daily (I did 4 cups over the past 2 weeks previously). I may even increase it more. I'm going to up my tea drinking and possibly add capsules. Need to see if tea or capsules are more potent. I've gotten this far and I'm going all in. Not that I wasn't before, but I'm not going to worry about what if it's lower. I'm only focused on making it bigger. ALL. IN.*

After that, I started drinking 3 cups of tea and 4 cups of bone broth daily. As you can see from my text, I was worried about what would happen if the scar thinned. Moving forward, my focus was on success, not worry or fear. I added in daily listening to a fear cleansing birth meditation. I upped my protein to 125 to 150 grams daily. I continued with my supplements, running, and massage. At this point, I was truly all in.

At about this same time, I hit a wall while on a 5-mile run. I went out to the Heritage Trail for a change of scenery and some motivation. I wanted so bad to walk but knew I couldn't quit. I remembered something from my breastfeeding days. *Never quit on your worst day.* I pushed through my 5 miles, and by the end, was picking up my pace and feeling good. It was just the reset I needed. The next few weeks were hot, but I got my 5-mile runs in, plus my smaller runs. I felt super strong.

For my 32-week appointment, I was back for another ultrasound at MFM. I was thrilled. They measured the thinnest spot as 2.9. I couldn't believe it. The MFM said, "your uterus looks strong." I told him about my bone broth. He couldn't believe it. He said he was going to tuck that away for future moms who need to strengthen their uterus. At this point, I was feeling good.

This was about the time I started my prenatal yoga class. Throughout my entire pregnancy, but even more committed at this point, I focused on the baby's position. I stood whenever possible. If I needed to sit for work, it was on a yoga/birth ball. I avoided couches as much as possible. Did tailor sitting on the floor, pelvic rocks, squats, kegels, and slept on my left side.

This was also about the time Braxton Hicks started. I wasn't surprised, given the introduction of the tea. With my rupture baby, Braxton Hicks started at the beginning of the third trimester, so these were a bit later to develop. I had them sporadically throughout the day and felt them a lot while I was running.

At my 34-week appointment, I was back with my OB, and she shared some surprising news. My MFM said that the range of my scar was 2.4 to 2.9 mm, and the 2.4 mm was never mentioned during my appointment. That 2.4 mm, again, had her worried. So, I'm thinking that I strengthened it, and her records are showing a .3 mm decrease in 2 weeks. We agreed that there was no need to make any decisions then, and we still had another ultrasound at 36 and 38 weeks. I just kept on my path, knowing the MFM said my uterus looked strong and assuming there is a fair amount of subjectivity in measuring, knowing they were measuring differently (abdominally vs. vaginally), and realizing a thin scar doesn't guarantee a rupture, just like a thicker scar doesn't make a labor risk-free of rupture.

At my 36-week appointment, my husband was able to attend. The plan was to do an ultrasound with our OB and then finalize a birth plan. We measured transvaginally with a full bladder and it ranged from 2.6 to 3.8. So, a tad smaller on the thin end and a tad bigger on the thick end from when she measured at 30 weeks. I was extremely pleased. Not knowing how much to expect it to thin, the fact that it maintained roughly the same thickness from 20 to 36 weeks was a huge win for me. Both Luke and I went into the actual appointment, ready for a trial of labor.

When the OB came in, she looked to us about what we were thinking. We could sense hesitation in her voice, but reviewed the literature, my stats, and told her that we felt comfortable proceeding with the plan. She quickly agreed, also saying that she discussed more with the radiologist who reviewed my ultrasound and reviewed the literature.

The radiologist thought 2 mm was an acceptable risk and my OB agreed that a trial of labor was reasonable.

We continued our discussion and addressed questions like when to come to the hospital, if other providers were supportive of the plan, the on-call schedule near my due date, concerns about electronic fetal monitoring, intentions for an all-natural labor, and more.

I'll pause here to say that heading into this appointment, Luke was nervous. I think he'd say that initially, this birth plan was not his first choice, but since the MFM and OB were okay with the plan, he'd be supportive as well. He really stepped up during this appointment, making sure we had all the information we wanted or needed, and talked through our concerns. It was clear, at that point, that he had fully transitioned and put his fears and worries aside to achieve this birth plan together. In hindsight, he didn't need the support of the MFM or OB to get there. It was great that we had a supportive team, but Luke is my number one cheerleader. He makes me a stronger and better person, and we did this together.

During that appointment, I had two unresolved concerns related to non-stress tests and cervical checks. Trying to be a reasonable patient and part of the team, I consented to a cervical check for that week (was 70% effaced, 1.5cm dilated, +3 station), but Luke told the OB that it was something we'd evaluate week by week, as I know cervical checks tell us nothing about when labor will start. I was not expecting a recommendation to start NSTs at 37 weeks. At the time, I didn't ask why, again, trying not to be unreasonable. Both Luke and I agreed that if anything was found on an NST, we'd evaluate our options then but didn't see a need to deny the NST right off the bat. We had a great discussion and all left feeling confident and good about the plan.

Following that appointment, I had some cramping and slight bleeding from the cervical check. I was so scared that labor was imminent and that I'd messed up my chances for a VBAR because of a cervical check. Luckily, it was temporary.

Another note here. Going back to my goals with this birth; I worked hard, with the guidance and help from my therapist, to come up with what would make this an ideal birth despite the delivery method. I came up with what I wanted or needed from this birth, how I wanted to feel, etc. We made contingency plans in case a c-section was needed, so that I could still have an ideal birth.

My 36th week of pregnancy was the first and only week of my pregnancy that I didn't get at least one 5-mile run in (I got 4.5 but ran out of time to finish). I got 19.55 running miles for the week, plus bonus walking miles. I knew what my next goal was for the next week.

My 37-week appointment consisted of the non-stress test, which checked out perfectly. I found out NSTs at 37 weeks are routine for this practice for anyone deemed advanced maternal age (which was me). My OB didn't ask for a cervical check at this appointment, which made me feel good about her as a provider.

On my 37th week of pregnancy, I was committed to getting my 5-mile-long run in and I did. The weather that week was extremely hot. During the work week, I got up and ran at a nearby track before work. On Saturday, June 12, the kids were invited to a friend's house for a play date. I did a late morning run while they played (this was one of the best runs; I got 4 miles in, and each mile was faster than the previous. It felt so good).

Luke decided to use that quiet time to read the Bradley book I had been asking him to read. He had not participated in the classes because he was always with the kids. He read chapters about emotional signposts of labor, dilation, and effacement. He read about back labor (which was incredibly useful with my labor). He read about the doctor's dilemma and ACOG's model of shared decision-making between doctor and patient. The Bradley book also talked about how oligohydramnios and failure to progress are two of the most common reasons noted for c-sections (even if not necessary). I think we will both always wonder where the OBs heart and intent were when he told us our first baby was facing brain damage or death but failed to share the risks of a c-section (that we remember. I'm sure he did, but we heard brain damage and death). Were we coerced or were we just naive? Either way, this was now our journey. We spent a lot of the afternoon talking about the birth plans, potential risks, what the doctors will be looking for, and how to decide when it's a true emergency (if there was one).

Not knowing we were under the clock, we put all the pieces together within a day of our baby's arrival.

Sunday, June 13. 37 weeks, 6 days. My mother-in-law came over for breakfast and I ate a huge, healthy breakfast (good thing, as that was my meal for the day, the way everything unfolded). My mother-in-law asked us about the timing of labor and when we would go to the hospital, about a 75-minute drive. I made the comment that I think the hardest part would be knowing the difference in Braxton Hicks and real labor. Luke looked at me, surprised I had been experiencing Braxton Hicks. Here I thought he knew, or just assumed he knew, that I was having Braxton Hicks, but he didn't. We talked about a few other labor-related things, including all the prep work I had done. My husband encouraged me to show her my squat. I did and she thought I was going to pop out a baby then and there, saying, "Get up or you're going to go into labor." Ha! Little did we know.

After my mother-in-law left, the kids got invited to my sister's house. I headed out for what would be my last run. By this time, it was 2 ish in the afternoon on a hot summer day (90 degrees plus humidity). This run was hard to push through. I needed 3 miles to get my goal of 20 miles for the week. I counted down the laps to 3 miles.

On the topic of running, after I ruptured, I questioned if I should have been running throughout that pregnancy and thought I had potentially put my baby at risk every time I ran. Then, the OB who assisted with the delivery and surgery said the fact that I ran so much was likely a contributing factor to why I had a good outcome, given our birth situation. That comment is what pushed me through my weekly runs. I needed this for my and my baby's health.

While I thoroughly enjoy running and love the self-challenge of running, my miles took me to new limits physically, mentally, and emotionally this pregnancy. I'll never forget my last week of runs with her in my belly. Anticipating her arrival. Enjoying the time with me, her, the sun, and music. The time to be intentional and thoughtful of breathing through every step or Braxton Hicks contraction.

I drank tons of water and Gatorade to make sure I stayed hydrated. I went to pick up the kids and that is probably when I first noticed some feelings that only came when I changed positions from sitting to standing, for example. We rushed to get the kids to soccer and didn't think anything of it.

At the soccer field, I could feel a tightening that wasn't a Braxton Hicks, but also would go away if I just changed from sitting to standing. Kept pushing fluids, assuming I was maybe dehydrated. With my previous two, I had lost my mucous plug three days before labor. I was expecting the same for this one and since I hadn't lost it yet, just assumed we were still, at least, a few days away from delivery.

When we got home, I told Luke something was up. It's certainly not labor, but now I was having sciatic nerve pain (not uncommon for me). I figured the baby was just dropping lower. Luke ran to the grocery store and while he was gone, I started noticing real contractions. They would start in my back and wrap low around my belly. These would happen whether I was sitting or standing. I timed my first one at about 8:45 pm. They were 10 to 20 minutes apart and inconsistent. I gave Luke the update, saying that this isn't labor yet. We have time.

Shortly after that, I had just the slightest tinged mucus. Putting all the clues together, that's when I knew this had the potential to be real. We decided it would be a good idea to have my mother-in-law come be with the kids, in case we needed to leave in the middle of the night. Once she arrived, Luke suggested we just head to the city with the hospital and could always get a hotel. That way, we weren't driving in the middle of the night, if necessary.

I agreed. We got packed up, including swimsuits for both of us and the kids because we thought we'd be at a hotel for the next few days and the kids could come swim. Ha!

We left home around 11:30 pm, getting potentially one last picture as a family of four (just in case). Contractions were more regular, but not close together or hard. My app told me that this is not consistent with labor, to consider eating, drinking, or resting to see if the pattern changes.

In the car, we put on the Rent soundtrack, talked, and sang the entire car ride. (This was the first chance I had to tell Luke what my ideal birth felt like, regardless of delivery and my formal birth plan). My contractions were getting closer together at this point, but easy to work through. We pulled into the city, needing to decide about where to go or what to do. Luke asked for a contraction update. Surprise! They are now every five minutes apart, but still not hard to work through. He had no idea contractions were getting closer. (Actually, I didn't either. I was diligent about putting them in the app but wasn't paying any attention to frequency.)

Now my app was saying this pattern is consistent with labor and we should call the doctor or hospital. So, we did, explaining if it wasn't for my birth history we would not be calling. Given my rupture, we thought we'd call and see what they wanted us to do.

The OB on call suggested we come in, saying she wouldn't admit us if it wasn't real labor. I was nervous. I did not want to be admitted if it wasn't real labor, and at this point, I was still hesitant. Yes, the timing would suggest real labor, but I knew it was early labor since they were so easy, and they hadn't been consistent for that long. Luke was sensitive to my concern as well. We agreed that we'd go get checked out, but also agreed we'd just go back to our original plan of a hotel if it wasn't real labor.

We checked in about 1:15 am on Monday, June 14, at 38 weeks to the day. The triage nurse got us hooked up to the NST and we did that for 20 minutes and confirmed that everything looked good. Since I was worried about the use of continuous fetal monitoring and how, sometimes, it can lead to unnecessary c-section, Luke asked the nurse to tell him what we are looking for. Our nurse was an NST educator and pulled up an example chart that looked good and one that didn't look good (no patient information on the chart). She also gave us scenarios that can look like an issue but are, in fact, common.

She then did a cervical check. I was 4 cm dilated. She then told us she would give the doctor an update, but she'd get us ready to be admitted. As she was talking to the doctor, I asked Luke if he could take pictures. I wanted to capture as much of this birth as possible. He then snapped a few pictures of me and us together. At this point, I was still all smiles, excited. I remembered in the Bradley book that if the emotional signpost was excited or happy, it was too early for the hospital (and the example in the book, being able to smile for a picture). I knew we had a while to go.

The nurse came back in with some news. The on-call doctor wasn't onboard with our birth plan. She was not convinced that I was in labor and said we needed to wait in triage for an hour and would monitor the NST and cervical change.

This was not part of the plan, and we thought we had addressed this with my OB. We didn't panic. We were fine waiting in triage and confident we wouldn't let this derail our plan. Our nurse was absolutely amazing. She kept coming in and adjusting the monitors, saying any missed contraction or heart tone could be a reason to question what's going on or suggest labor wasn't progressing safely. She was truly a patient advocate.

At about 3 am, our additional hour was up. I progressed to 5 cm dilated and the nurse let us know the doctor would be in to discuss the plan. The doctor entered the triage room and jumped right into her clearly prepped dissenting speech. A quick intro of her name and then a long explanation about how she is an OB who is medically trained for high-risk situations, that the governing body (ACOG) does not recommend a trial of labor after a rupture, etc. Once she got done, Luke politely shared all the reasons we were comfortable with proceeding. He reasoned with her and took the time to help her understand everything we've done to prepare for this. Luke was a huge advocate. Hard to believe the transformation he went through and the commitment to me that he could turn what was once huge fears into something he could argue better than me, on behalf of me. It was a defining moment for this birth and for our relationship. His commitment was truly on display.

Honestly, I didn't engage in the discussion at all. I did not want to lose focus on what I was there to do: labor and have a baby. I knew if I got distracted, it could do all sorts of things to labor. By then, I was starting to focus on my contractions, which were getting a little more intense. Plus, I would have been less diplomatic about her recommendation and said, "thanks but I'm not interested in your opinion."

Luke's approach was extremely helpful and persuasive. By the end, the doctor and Luke were exchanging a bit of personal history. He was able to level with her so whatever risk she posed was completely dismissed. We were on our way to being admitted.

Here's a couple things to note here:

I was Group Strep B positive, and she said she was comfortable getting an IV started and guaranteeing 4 hours of uninterrupted, intervention-free labor. (Perfect; we all got what we wanted.)

The doctor's shift was over at 8 am and my OB would start her shift.

We thought her strategy was to admit us, and hopefully, not have to do anything before shift change.

At about 3:25am, we left triage and headed to our labor and delivery room. I had one hard contraction in the hallway on the 20-foot walk to our room. It was like a movie scene, bent over in the hallway on the guardrail. I was certain the nurses and on-call doctor were judging me. She is a 5, so how is she going to make it without any interventions? Oh well.

We entered our room, and our nurse prepped the bed. While she did that, I had a contraction on the toilet. I wiped and saw no mucous plug, no bloody show, nothing but clear urine. I thought that we were in for a long night.

I got up off the toilet and had an immediate contraction and it was strong. I got down on all fours on the bathroom floor. The time was 3:28 am.

The nurse asked Luke if my water broke, which it had not. Both agreed that things were ramping up quickly and we should get ready for a baby sooner than later. The nurse called for nursing help and said I needed to get to the bed.

I got there. Had one contraction on my back that I could barely handle. Back on my hands and knees on the bed. It's crazy to me how your body just knows what position to get in.

Luke, having read the Bradley book, started applying deep pressure to my sacrum, which felt amazing.

Contractions were coming hard and fast. In my mind, we still had hours to go. I was starting to doubt if I could handle this for several more hours. I questioned how I did a natural labor last time and specifically how I got so relaxed. See, with my prior birth, I had plenty of time to get relaxed, work with each contraction, and let my body go loose. This time, there was no way I could relax, much less sleep through this.

I asked if it was too late for an epidural, saying that I wasn't sure if I could do this. The nurse said it wasn't too late, but Luke, being the awesome Bradley coach he was, said this was the self-doubt stage, which means I'm close to meeting our baby. Another nurse jumped in and backed Luke up, agreeing that the baby would be here soon. I knew they were right, but still in disbelief. This labor was intense, but I did not want an epidural messing up my chance at a VBAR.

At 3:48 am, I started involuntarily pushing. At that time, the other nurse got right in my face and helped me get my breathing under control. I think I did get control and was able to work with labor rather than against it. She walked away for a second and I said I needed her back telling me when and how to breathe. I'm so thankful for her coaching. Luke continued with the counter pressure on my back.

At 3:49 am, my water broke. No artificial rupture of membranes! Sometime after that, Luke said the doctor came flying into the room, gloving up on the run. Another movie scene, Luke said a nurse swung a stool under her as she was sitting down. She said after the current contraction was over, and I should flip over, which I did. Luke said that when I flipped, he could already see the baby's head crowning. The doctor said, "Let's have a baby!" Two contractions and 6 pushes later, our baby was born at 3:59 am.

What followed was pure bliss. Immediate skin to skin, no wiping of our baby, right to me. Delayed cord clamping, which I got to cut (I almost cut the doctor's finger instead of the cord). The nurses grabbed Luke's phone and got photos that completely captured the emotions of me and Luke.

I can't describe what was going through my mind. Triumph, victory, success, relief, healthy, safe, here. With those two pushing contractions,

I talked to my baby and body. We can do this. We are so close. I had full faith and trust in God.

We did it. I knew all along we would. It was so, so perfect. Everything about it. I think that when I reflect on the best parts of this birth, it will be the tears of joy on Luke's face right after she was born. I remember experiencing a birth high with my second baby and Luke, and I had this incredible bonding experience. This was more than a birth high and what Luke and I had ventured on together was more than bonding. This experience took our relationship to a new level, truly becoming and acting as one to bring this new human into the world. Nothing can accurately describe our journey and the emotions that came with it.

When I say we did it, I mean it. It took me and Luke, together as one team. Also, my MFM and his clinic team. My OB. The nursing staff. My Bradley instructor. My birth therapist. Our couple's counselor. Support and prayers from family and friends. Promising birth stories from other moms. Faith and trust in God. Each had an important and necessary role. It truly took a village. It was hard work and dedication, but it paid dividends.

I had minor lacerations in the vaginal wall. No symptoms of uterine rupture. I held our baby for a long time, and put her to breast right away, in which she latched perfectly. I'm not even sure how long I held her before deciding she could get weighed. She didn't leave our room for the first 24 hours.

My MFM was the first one to round on me after delivery. I cried when I thanked him for his support, going beyond ACOG's recommendation and truly hearing and seeing my needs and wants for this birth. He was an integral part of this journey for us and gives me hope in a better way of maternal-fetal health.

He said I've become an expert and people need to hear my story; it has the power to change lives. I'm not sure what this means yet, but I'm starting by sharing my birth story. I'll be thinking about how I can help change the narrative of maternal and fetal medicine.

He also said something so inspiring to me. He explained that he sees a lot of hard things in his work, but it's my story, and others like mine, that inspire him to continue doing what he's doing. That alone gives me so much hope for our maternal-fetal health system.

When I was discharged, it was a new OB from the practice doing rounds that day. I was up, holding baby when she came in the room. She said something along the lines of the one who had us all worried; "Here you stand with your baby." I understand the fear providers have. I know they see a lot of scary things. I was one of those scary things four years earlier. However, I spent the last four years planning and working towards this birth and these moments. Below is a saying that I looked at and read every day for the last four years:

> *And one day she discovered that she was fierce, and strong, and full of fire, and that not even she could hold herself back because her passion burned brighter than her fears.*

I think that's what I did on this journey. I've learned a lot the past 4 years, but also the last 10 months. The power of mind-body connection, and power of prayer and trust in God is not lost on me. Here are some things that may be obvious to some, but became apparent to me:

What we feed our body makes a difference.

How we exercise, work, relax, stretch, treat our body makes a difference.

Who we surround ourselves with can largely impact our choices and decisions.

Our thoughts can change our future.

We can do amazing things when we put our mind and body at work together.

Listen and trust your intuition. It's a powerful thing.

Most importantly, remember the power of prayer and trust in God. I say all of this knowing I did everything in my power to make this happen, but ultimately, it was in God's hands. Complete faith and trust in God.

Brianna – VBAC

1st Baby

Born June 2018, at 40 + 4. I was induced because of lack of fluid. The baby was no longer making urine and had reduced movements. The baby was posterior asynclitic. At 7 pm, the balloon catheter inserted and removed the next morning at 7 am, and I was dilated 3 cm. I commenced Syntocin drip at 9:30, as I did not contact. The Syntocin dose increased over the day. Around 3pm, things started to go downhill. I was getting five contractions in a row, without a break. I had gas and Remi-fentanyl, but nothing helped. My bubs heart rate kept dipping. Got an epidural at 5:30 pm to see if this would relax myself and bubs. By the time the epidural was in, and I was being wheeled to theatre for foetal distress, I was still only 3 cm dilated. I had an emergency caesar, where they found that bubs was obstructed due to poor positioning. Epidural was topped up for the caesar but turned into a T1 block (blocked from my shoulders down). I had a loss of consciousness for 3.5 hours due to extremely low BP from epidural. I missed out on those first few hours of cuddles with my son and had some nerve damage to my sacral area.

2nd Baby

Born 5/6/2020, 41+4During my initial consult with my OB, I expressed some desire to have a VBAC if my baby was in the right position. I said I didn't want to be induced, and it was suggested that I would have an RSC (elective caesarean) at 42 weeks if I hadn't gone into labor. My doctor said I was a great candidate for a VBAC.

After this, there was no further discussion about the delivery until my 40-week appointment. I started researching VBAC articles, stats, and reading all the stories on [this page].

In order to avoid this baby-turning posterior, I only slept on a side and sat upright or forward on the couch.

» 34 weeks, I began spinning babies, remedial massage, chiro, and began a calm birth course.

- » 36 weeks, I started raspberry leaf tea.
- » 38 weeks, I commenced acupressure and acupuncture.
- » 40 weeks, I commenced breast pumping 2 to 3 times a day.

During my 40-week appointment, my OB states that he was beginning to doubt whether this baby would come out vaginally, as my baby was measuring 50 weeks. He said, "what do you want to do?" I was gutted. I felt like my body was letting me down and that my OB and I weren't on the same page. I was told during my previous pregnancy that my son was "enormous" and he was only 7lbs, 13oz.

Once I hit 40 weeks, all of a sudden, the OBs got stressed. They told me that I was measuring 50 weeks at my 40-week appt. I was also told that, as I hadn't delivered at 40 weeks, that it was "unlikely" that I would achieve my VBAC. It was insinuated that I should have a cessation but not directly put to me. I had an appointment scheduled for me of a Friday. My OB doesn't see antenatal patients on a Friday morning. I called the hospital to see if he had a theatre list that afternoon. They said yes. The hospital said I had called. He thought I was in labour, so he called me. I told him I wasn't in labour, but I had called to see if he had a Friday afternoon theatre list, to see if he was earmarking me for a caesar. After that, he stepped back and let me do my thing. I delivered a week and a half later.

I said I wasn't going to be induced or have a caesar at this point because I was "due," not "overdue," and people birth big babies all the time. I also said that I don't have GD and bubs HR, fluid and movements were all fine, so there was no medical reason to intervene. He hesitated but agreed. I left the appointment angry and deflated and started doing everything I could to induce myself naturally, including breast pumping. Later that week, I lost my mucous plug and had some Braxton Hicks. It didn't eventuate to anything.

At my 41-week appointment, I told my doctor that my new plan was to have a balloon and an AROM at 42 weeks. If unsuccessful, I would have an RSC. He was hesitant but agreed.

At 41 + 1, I began early spontaneous labor. This became 2 days of spurious labour with bladder spasms, as I couldn't urinate properly. I hadn't slept for 2 days and could barely eat. So, I went into hospital at midnight to be reviewed by my OB. Mentally, I was preparing myself for a caesarean. I was 3 cm dilated, so I had an AROM. Then, I was able to wee (thank God). From there on, my contractions were smoother and ramped up. At 6:30 am, I was 4 cm dilated but I requested an epidural (which was not part of my plan). The epidural was amazing! I ended up having a 30-minute sleep. I woke up, as I was 8 cm dilated. At 11am, it was time to start pushing. By 12 pm, my bubs HR was getting elevated. I consented to forceps in theatre, and out she came! I bawled my eyes out. I couldn't believe that I did it. I felt like everyone had written me off beforehand. It was the most empowering feeling.

She was 9lbs, 6oz, with a 37cm head circumference.

I had an episiotomy and quite a bit of stitching to the front of me, but the recovery is already so much easier than a caesarean.

I got to hold my baby girl as soon as she was born. It was so magical!

I am currently 24 weeks pregnant with my 3rd.

Brianna Edmonston, Victoria, Australia

Hannah – VBAC with GDM

This is the story I wrote in the hours after my 2nd VBAC baby was born to share with the VBAC group. Super proud of myself and my baby working together. I was up against it with GDM and high BMI of 40, and a hospital transfer late in my pregnancy.

2nd VBAC: Surprise gender, induction by breaking waters with pushy doctor

Background 2012: Waters broke at home. 41+3 with first. I was already booked for induction that day, so I was told to come in. My drip started and then I asked for every drug available. The cascade of drugs, I believe, is the reason it ended in caesarean.

2015: 41 weeks, my spontaneous labour lasted 6 hours, and was a drug-free VBAC with vacuum delivery. There was some tearing and a PPH of 1 litre, but it still felt awesome afterwards and I didn't need transfusion.

2021: I found out I was pregnant in May 2020, so it was right in the middle of lockdown in Melbourne.

My first appointment was a phone appointment with a midwife who recommended I get an early GDM test, as I had a high BMI of close to 40. They also said they would bring me up in a meeting. There's a technical term for it but I can't remember what the meeting is called. It was decided that I should take blood thinners, as my higher BMI could mean my placenta and cord might not function correctly and the baby might end up with restricted growth. In the same breath, I was also told that I would need to have growth scans at 28, 32, and 36 weeks, due to my BMI and fear of a large baby. After consideration, I decided against the blood thinners.

I ended up putting off the early glucose test until about 22 weeks and it came back fine. Though the routine 28-week check came back 0.5 over. A meeting was arranged with the diabetes educator and a phone call with a dietician. I was rushed through the education session, as they had double booked my first face-to-face appointment with the midwives, so I left feeling quite anxious about the whole GDM thing, but I picked it up quickly and worked out a good diet that kept my numbers well below where they needed to be.

At my first meeting with one of the obstetricians (small country hospital so no option for continued care; you just get who you get), she said, "you've got GDM. You best go to the metropolitan hospital 30 mins away, because you'll most likely end up on insulin and end up there anyway." I said, "No, thanks. I would like to see how I go." In the same conversation, she weighed me, checked my BMI, and said, "You're going to go over on your BMI so you should probably just go to the metropolitan hospital, because you're going to put on weight and end up there anyway." I just sat there and waited for her to talk. She told me to come back in 4 weeks and we'll re-evaluate. Four weeks later, and I had lost half a kilo. I wished so bad that the obstetrician would be on that day, but she wasn't.

So, my care continued with the country hospital until about 37 weeks, where they had a major issue in their theatre and couldn't take any maternity patients and the ward was closed. They said, "It will be back up by the time you're 40 weeks." It was not. So, the hospital I had fought so hard to have my baby at and the same hospital I had my previous 2 babies at, 1 VBAC, could no longer take me, and I had to transfer to the metropolitan hospital.

From there, I received great care and had the head midwife call me to introduce herself. At 41 weeks, we headed in for induction (which I didn't want), only to be told once I was there that they had a big influx, so I could go home until they called me to come back. They called at 41+4. I went in and had my water broke but said no to the Syntocinon drip. Overall, between the two hospitals, no one ever said I couldn't have a VBAC, but I fought a lot to try and stay at the smaller hospital and just kept hearing "hospital policy." It was a completely different experience, having appointments and a baby during a pandemic. If it was my first baby, it would've impacted my mental health but knowing that the level of care wasn't the normal standard, somehow, managed to get me through it.

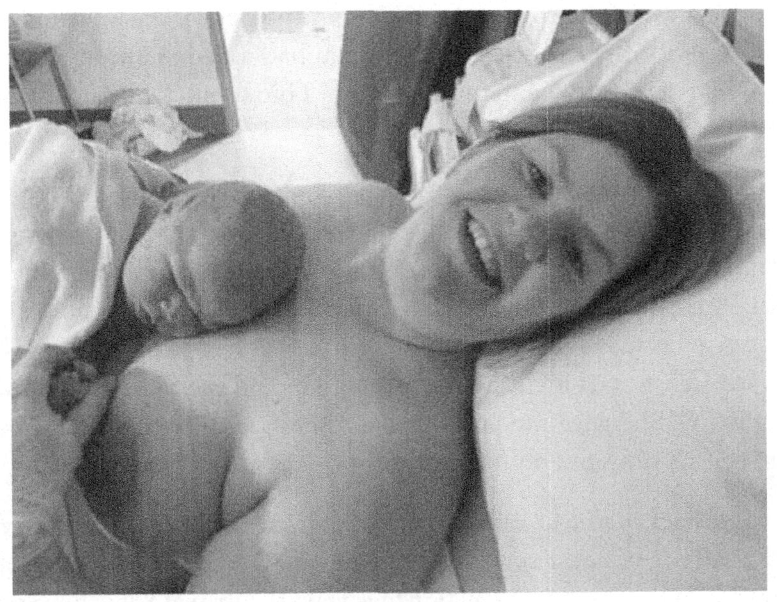

Parker William Archer @ 41+4
(diet controlled GDM)
23/01/21 @10:03pm
4.165kg
HC 36.5
Hannah Archer, Victoria, Australia

Our lockdown baby was due 12/01/21. At 36 weeks, I found out my chosen hospital had to close its ward due to a theatre issue. So, I had to switch to a hospital 3 times further away but with slightly relaxed rules on my GDM diet controlled and how far they would let me go over. I had monitoring done 3 times over the 11 days I was over. Each time, my baby was happy, so they let me go a little longer. They decided that they would try to induce me by breaking my waters at some point over the weekend but had to wait for the call to say the hospital had a bed. Saturday, 23rd, at 41+4, we got a call; "Be in here in an hour." I burst into tears, a combination of fear and excitement.

We arrived on the birth suite at 1:30 pm and I was hooked up to get a trace on the baby before breaking waters. Bubs was moving around a lot and had an elevated heart rate. We had to wait 2 hours for it to calm down. Finally, at 4 pm, the midwife broke my waters. The doctor came in because I refused the Syntocinon drip and asked, "How long do you want before we start it?" I said, "3 to 4 hours," and she said, "I'll be back in an hour." She gave me an hour and a half, and in that time, I had small contractions but nothing serious.

She came back in at 5:30, and I asked to be given until 6. She didn't come back at all after that. I continued having small contractions until 7:30, where my midwife said, "Why don't we start the drip at 8 low dose and see what happens?" She said, "Let's just hope something happens before then." I was okay with this, as I felt like I trusted her judgement better than the pushy doctor.

You couldn't write what happens next. From the moment we made the plan, I start contracting 3 times every 10 minutes. They're super intense and fast. My midwife was practically dancing around the room, and I would've if I could've. About 9, she asked if I wanted to try the shower and I said, yes. I got in there, had 1 contraction, and said, "I need to push." She said, "Okay, let's check out what's going on." A cervical check showed that I was only 6 cm, but she said, "Don't worry, it won't take long." Just before 9:30, there was a shift change, and I was sad that she was going to miss the birth but so thankful she advocated for me and gave my body time.

So, I'm meeting my new midwife and student MW at the same time as I'm trying not to push but half pushing. My new midwife suggested a wee might do good to bring the baby's head down once my bladder was empty. So, I waddled to the toilet at about 9:45 pm (less than an hour after I was told I was 6 cm), contracting the whole way. I tried to wee but couldn't. I started to push instead. It just took over my body. The midwife was trying to get me to lean back so she could work out if the baby was coming, I said that I can't a few times. So, I got stern and said, "We need to be able to catch the baby," so my husband practically dragged me out of the bathroom back beside the bed.

They placed a mat under me and said, "Go for it." I could feel his head coming down and pushed. The midwife placed a warm compress on my perineum. I could feel the ring of fire. She said that I needed little pushes to get the nose out and I felt his head come out. I still had the contraction, so she said, "push again," and most of his body was out. She went to say, "One more little push," but he just slid out. She said, "Open up your legs so I can pass him through." Him? Is it a boy? I took him and checked for myself, and said to my husband, "Oh my God, it's a boy." We both felt it was a girl and were both gobsmacked.

They helped me up on to the bed, where we had delayed cord clamping and my hubby cut the cord. They did manual removal of my placenta and checked my blood loss, as I had a PPH with my first VBAC. I only lost around 150 mls this time, and best of all, no tears; just a graze but I copped some nasty haemorrhoids. I was up within an hour or so having a shower. I stayed for about 20 hours after his birth and took off home, so our older two could find out if they had a brother or sister.

It was an amazing way to finish off our family.

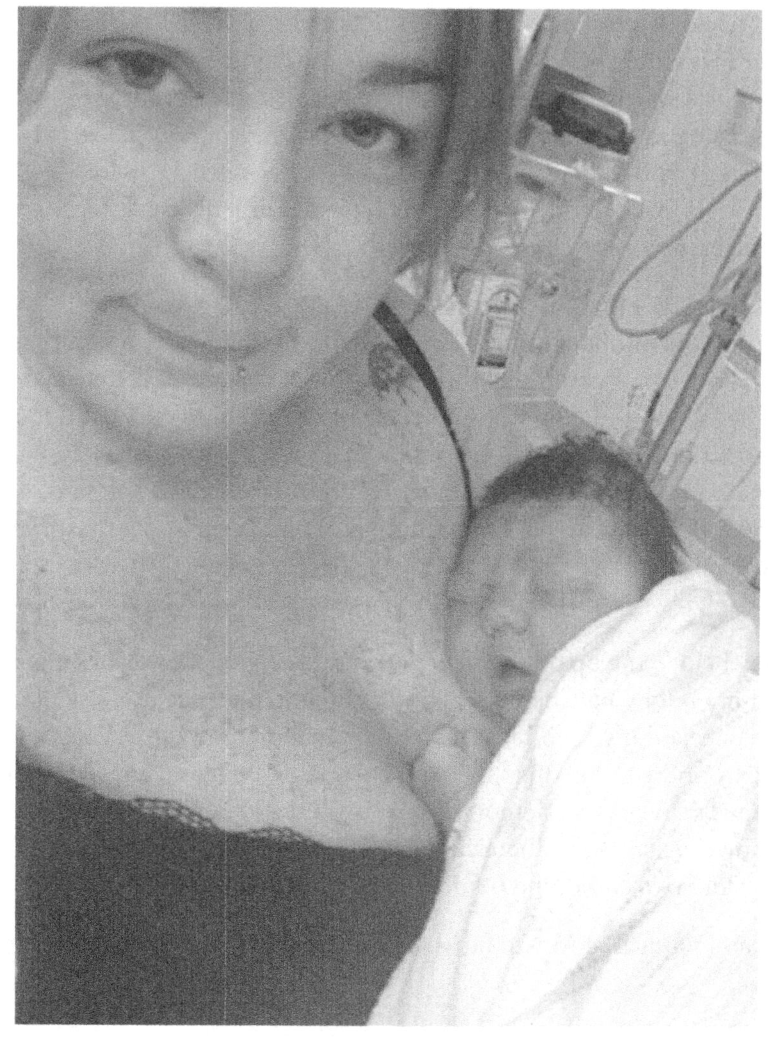

Jordon Betham, NSW, Australia

Jordon – VBAC

My name is Jordon, and I had a VBAC that fit into the high BMI range.

After I had my first born, I was broken, ashamed, and disappointed in myself, my body, and my care providers.

Once I pulled myself out of the darkness of postnatal depression, I was determined that I would never ever feel so disempowered again.

So it began, my VBAC journey. I had reached out amongst fellow women and trained professionals to absorb all that I could to give myself the best possible chance. The unified response was, "You can 100% achieve a VBAC."

Armed with knowledge, feeling empowered and determined to boot, I went into my booking appointment. The midwife informed me that, due to my previous cesarean and high BMI, I would need to book in to see the doctors for some of my appointments but assured me that I had every chance of having the birth I wanted.

Prior to my first appointment with one of the doctors, I attended a NBAC group. We all shared our stories, we all cried, and there was a unified feeling in the room. We all wanted a positive birth experience, regardless of how that looked.

Here I was, feeling even more supported than I had ever imagined. Then, I saw the OB.

From the moment she walked me into the room, she had decided that, regardless of what I said or did, she would be scheduling me in for a cesarean. The idea of a water birth had well and truly flown out the window in a hospital setting, and I was too scared something would go wrong if we tried to have a home birth.

I went home after every appointment, crying my eyes out after hearing on repeat, "Your previous c-section, previous big baby, and your high BMI mean you shouldn't try for a VBAC because you and your baby might die."

At one stage, I recall her calling in the register after I went off at her because she had told me, in no uncertain terms, that I was putting my baby at risk and was going to kill them.

Needless to say, I asked to NEVER see her again.

The next OB must have been warned about the overreactive woman who was refusing recommendations, I told her politely that I didn't have the 3rd trimester growth scan because I knew my baby would be big (my husband is a 6'4 Samoan/Polish man and I'm a muscly 5'11 Australian), and I wouldn't be turning up to a scheduled c-section.

She took the time to hear me, she could see I had educated myself and was making an informed decision, and we came to the agreement that I would be scheduled for induction at 40 weeks and 11 days.

40 weeks and 10 days comes around. I hadn't seen a midwife since my NBAC group – just doctors and the doula we had felt connected to had ghosted us. I had worked myself up into a state; I had an induction last time and it was awful. I didn't want that again. Why couldn't something—anything—happen naturally?

Then, it did, like a freight train.

Contractions began at 3 pm, after losing my mucus plug in the morning, I walked through them for an hour, bounced on an exercise ball for 2 hours, and then hopped into the shower. By 7 pm, they were 3 mins apart and 1 min long. A quick call to birth unit and we were on our way.

I had a vaginal exam at around 8 pm and was 4 cm dilated. I can't explain how empowered I felt, just getting to this point. I kept repeating, in my mind, all the positive things I had read about achieving VBACs.

The pain was excruciating across my back, position changes weren't helping, and I needed gas. I agreed to a vaginal exam at 10 pm and I was almost fully dilated but the baby was posterior.

Despite being a busy night with 8 women, all in well-established labour, the midwives had read my notes carefully and knew how badly I wanted a VBAC.

They spoke to me kindly and directly with all the information. If I really wanted a VBAC, the best chance I had would be to get an epidural and episiotomy so that they could turn the baby slightly, so that the baby could get through my pelvis.

I was making a choice that needed to be right for me, something I felt that I had the information for, and would be a positive experience.

I agreed and signed the paperwork to go ahead. In the meantime, I contorted against contractions; I was terrified that my baby might get stuck if I contracted them down into my pelvis while posterior (and presumably big).

11:30 pm rolled around, the epidural was in, episiotomy performed, and baby turned. Every single person in that room was supporting me in getting this VBAC.

Time to push!

Boy, did I push! It was my niece's birthday the following day and, as trivial as it was, I wanted the baby to have their own birthday.

Sure enough, 15 mins of hard pushing and our beautiful little, well, 4.3kg, baby girl had arrived into the world via VBAC.

I burst into tears and said, "I did it! I bloody did it!"

I will never be able to express exactly how the VBAC made me feel or how grateful I am towards the midwives who looked after me. It changed my life, but what I can tell you is that I got my VBAC because I felt empowered. Regardless of my previous birth or my weight, there was a great big community out there, throwing their support towards me.

My VBAC has changed so much for me and, in all honesty, has inspired me to change my career. I am currently a student midwife and love supporting women in their journeys.

Unfortunately, I was too inwardly focused to think about photos during the birth, but this was taken almost immediately after.

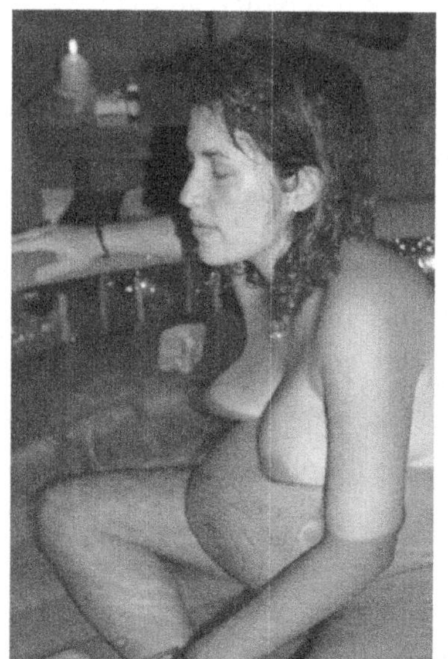

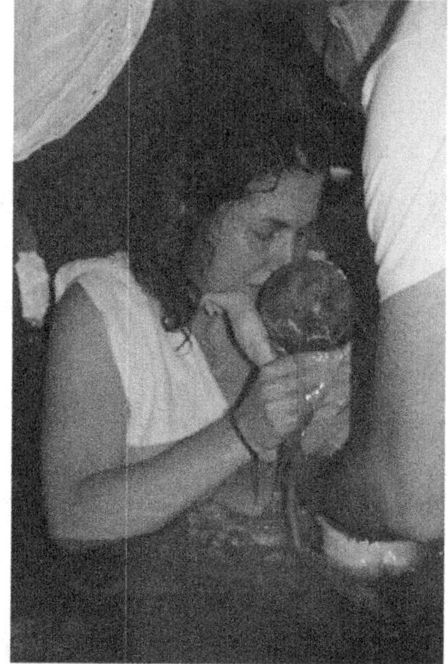

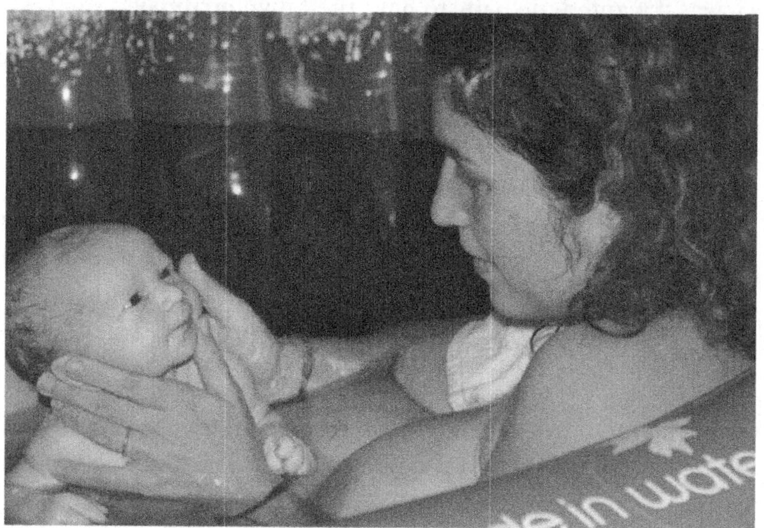

Erin Quinn, NSW Australia

Erin – Homebirth after 2 Caesareans

The HBA2C Birth of Samara

My first two daughters were both born by caesarean. The first was a classic failure to progress, or failure to wait. I planned a homebirth with my second, but after four days of labour, my waters broke with thick meconium. I transferred to hospital, labour stalled, and after several hours, the baby started to show signs of distress. They were both big babies. They both went from more favourable to less favourable positions during labour or shortly before. Neither of them ever engaged in my pelvis. I thought my body was truly a lemon. I could blame the hospital for my first surgery, but after my second surgery, when I had planned a homebirth and completely trusted the process, I felt the buck stopped with me. I had failed.

I wanted a third child, but I was scared to conceive again. I was scared that I wanted another chance to birth naturally, instead of another baby. I was scared of going through the whole emotional journey again, only to fail again. Samara got tired of waiting for me to work it out; her conception was a happy surprise for us. I planned a homebirth. Of course, I did. I don't have it in me to choose caesarean. I believe the way we are born matters. Deep in my soul, I knew what birth was supposed to be like. I had to try again, though, for the first time, I had no belief in my body. I was lucky enough to be able to surround myself with three wonderful women—two midwives and a doula—who did all the believing for me.

It was an emotional pregnancy, not knowing if the birth was going to be my life's high or low point. I cut out sugar from my diet, and as much processed food as I could, though I fell off the wagon at Christmas. I did techniques from Spinning Babies every day to balance my pelvis. My husband bought me a rebozo and we started using it. In third trimester, I began having Bowen therapy and acupuncture to optimise my pelvis. I had warm baths and talked to my baby, asking her to help me birth her beautifully. Even my 3-year-old started saying, "move down, baby." At my 35-week prenatal visit, my midwife announced that my baby was slightly engaged. I promptly burst into tears and asked if she was lying.

It was such a huge moment for me. I had seriously wondered if there was some kind of physical barrier preventing my babies from entering the pelvis. But there she was! Maybe I could do this? Maybe my body wasn't broken?

When I was 39+5, I felt the first tightening on a Monday night, while in bed. Nothing too bad, I was able to simply breathe through them. I felt a bit teary. I was afraid that I was going to be in labour for days again, and I didn't want to send my kids away. They were going to stay with my parents. As much as I love the idea of siblings at a birth, for this birth, I felt the only one who needed mothering was me. Now that the time was imminent, I didn't want to say goodbye to them. I think they picked up on it; my 2-year-old was restless, and my 3-year-old ended up joining us in bed. The tightening stopped once I got up for the day, increasing again towards evening. I expected that I was going to have a few nights of prelabour, as I had with my others. I sent my husband off to his piano lesson. He insisted I text my birth support people. I sent a message to the effect that I was having contractions, but tonight wasn't going to be the night.

As soon as I tried to go to bed, the contractions notched up. I quickly realised I wasn't going to be able to rest and decided to have a bath by candlelight. I laboured there for a while, just watching the flames. I tried again to go to bed, still in denial, and then ended up in the shower. I was banging on the wall, counting myself through the surges. I quickly changed it to banging on my own thigh, worried I was going to wake the kids. I began to think that I might need my doula there, but I could't call out. My husband read my mind, because he came to check on me and suggested he call her.

When Nat arrived, I was kneeling against the lounge and moaning into the cushions. Later, Nat told me that she could hear me from the street. She asked why we hadn't filled the pool or called the midwives. She proceeded to do so. I heard her say, "She's vocalising quite strongly."

The pool got set up and I got in. Instant relief! I spent most of the time in a kneeling position, leaning over the side. I tried some other positions, because I thought that maybe I should, but I realised that the position I had chosen instinctively was the most comfortable one for me. I held on to loving hands through the contractions. I started off deliberately keeping my hands loose, but at some point, that strategy was abandoned. I stayed in the pool, moaning through surges, and sleeping in between. Everyone was quiet and just held the space for me. I was aware of how present and supportive they were. It helped so much, even though no one was doing anything. I thought I was going to need a lot of guidance and cheerleading, but I didn't. At some point, I was aware of soft voices. I wanted to tell them they didn't need to whisper, but I couldn't. Almost from the first contraction, I had entered a trancelike state. In the pool, I was in my own little world, in this state, where I was aware of my surroundings but separate from them. I had random thoughts that I wanted to voice, but in my trance, I couldn't verbalise. One of the only things I managed to say was, "I can't do this for four days." Everyone assured me this was not going to last for four days, that I was in real, strong, active labour.

My husband called my parents. They arrived just as my 2-year-old woke up at 5:30. The kids transferred easily from bed to car, with some sleepy glances my way. My mum briefly poked her head into the lounge room to smile at me. After the girls were safely on their way with their grandparents, someone suggested I go for a walk before the sun came up. I didn't want to get out of the pool, but I recognised that we were in a lull, and I certainly didn't want to leave the house in daylight. Somehow, I did get out of the pool and into a nightie. Dan and Nat accompanied me around the block. I remember Nat asking if we got opossums, and Dan mentioned the local bat colony. I was vaguely disappointed that we didn't see any bats that morning. I was feeling a bit sulky, thinking of how tired I was, and that if labour was stalled, I wanted it to stop altogether so I could sleep. In hindsight, this was probably transition. Still, I wasn't believing that this baby was really going to come without help. Nat was encouraging me to walk through contractions, but I kept stopping and moaning into Dan's shoulder. The block seemed enormous to me. We got to the top of our street and our house looked like it was miles away. I finally decided to woman up and walk through the contractions. I think I was just so eager to get back home.

I laboured in the toilet for a while. I remember this time as being the hardest part. The contractions were coming harder and faster, and I was finding it difficult to rally myself enough for the next one. I reached down and I felt my baby's head, behind a bulging bag of waters, just a few centimetres inside me. Dan felt it too, and it was the most wonderful, intimate thing to be touching our unborn baby together. That was the first inkling I had that I might be about to birth a baby vaginally. I moved into the pool again, but the contractions slowed right down, so I went back to the toilet. I was being encouraged to stay upright, and someone brought a step for me to put one leg up, but the contractions were too intense for me to integrate this way. I dropped to all fours again, where I could surrender to the surges instead of fighting against them. Dan pointed out that the contractions were further apart in this position, and I said something rude to him.

Her head did get lower, against all my expectations. Someone said it was time to move back into the pool, and I didn't think I could, after all that. The few metres between toilet and pool seemed like an insurmountable distance, but with everyone's help and coaxing, I managed to get back in. I don't remember much of this time. I remember being unable to avoid blowing bubbles during the surges. I remember being told to push. It was only then that I realised that the enormous pressure I had been feeling at the peak of every contraction for quite some time was a pushing urge. It wasn't what I had expected. I expected it to be involuntary, a relief and a release, as I had heard it described. Instead, I felt it as quite a scary, splitting sensation, that I did NOT want to push through. I couldn't. I just wanted to breathe through it. I pretended to push. I asked if my vagina was about to be ruined, and everyone assured me it wouldn't be. They got me into a supported squat and prepared me to catch my baby. I said I wanted Dan to catch her. Reaching down seemed impossible to me, and I wanted him to have the honour anyway. He wanted me to catch her, and we argued about it for a minute. In the end, we both caught her.

There was no ring of fire. I didn't realise, when her head came out, it was just a continuation of the splitting sensation I was already feeling. I remember the sensation of her shoulders rotating. I said something like,

"Ooh, stop it, baby," and someone explained what was happening. Then she was out. It was 8:30 am. My waters broke as she emerged in her caul. I saw her eyes wide open, looking straight at me from under the water as I lifted her out. The cord was short. I couldn't bring her up to my chest as I wanted to. She didn't cry, but she was making little gurgling noises. I was encouraged to rub her back and blow into her face. I wasn't worried. She seemed present to me, and she was fine.

I thought I would have a huge outpouring of emotion when she was born. I wanted to have that "I did it!" moment, but I think I was just too overwhelmed. Finally having the natural birth I had always dreamed of, but never thought I would get, my whole world and self-identity shifted, and it was too much to process in a moment. I just calmly inhaled my baby. At the time of writing, she is 8 months old, and I have "I did it!" moments every day. It was so wonderful to have the joy of a new baby unadulterated, without the accompanying grief of an ungentle birth. I cried so often when my older kids were babies. This time, the only sadness I have experienced is that I will never get to experience real birth again. It was unquestionably the most amazing experience of my life. It wasn't painless, nor technically orgasmic, but it was ecstatic. The contractions hurt, but I wasn't suffering, or unable to cope. Birthing uninterrupted, feeling safe and supported, and allowing my hormones to work exactly as they were supposed to, I entered a primal place where the pain was not bigger than me. I feel like I've discovered the secret of the universe, and I could do it again and again. How heartbreaking it is to discover this just as our family is complete! How exquisite it would have been to know this secret on the day I became a mother for the first time!

My chequered birth history reawakened my childhood interest in becoming a midwife. After my first caesarean, I immediately started planning my VBAC. I went to see a homebirth midwife to see if I was a good candidate for HBAC, and I cried to her that day that I wanted to become a midwife, but I couldn't if I had never had a vaginal birth. She did reassure me that being a good midwife had more to do with empathy than experiencing vaginal birth (and I know this is true), but I don't know that I ever would have been able to put aside my grief and my impostor syndrome to truly be with women.

Having a VBAC did not change the past or alleviate the sadness around my caesarean births. If anything, I was more acutely aware of what my first babies and I missed out on. But it was healing. It healed me of feeling like less of a woman, of feeling broken and incapable. It truly changed my sense of self and hence, my life. Now, I am a student midwife, and I would not have taken this step if I hadn't had a VBAC.

Siobhan – VBAC with ECV for Breech

Caesarean birth, September 2016 – My first was pregnancy was textbook until he was found to be footling breech at 36 weeks. We tried to turn him via ECV. It was excruciating and unsuccessful. They said, "You can try again, but it probably won't work." I was immediately given a form, which at the time, I was a bit confused about what it was: signing consent to a caesarean. I was devastated but continued with the caesarean, as much as I did not want to do it. I thought that once I had signed the form, I could not back out. I was heartbroken for the birth that I had hoped for. I was told on a few occasions that I would be a good candidate for a VBAC if we wanted more children. We did want more children. I then began researching before my son was born. The physical recovery from surgery was good, but the emotional recovery was not good; I felt entirely disempowered. Following my son's birth, I had postnatal anxiety. We also had many breastfeeding issues. I was determined to overcome these as I was not going to have another experience taken from me. I usually am one to stand my ground for what I think is right, so this experience shook me.

VBAC, November 2018 – With our second pregnancy, I was determined that I would be having a VBAC, despite the many comments; "I didn't think they would allow you to do that" and "isn't that dangerous?" If my pregnancy was anything like my last, it would be smooth, and I couldn't possibly have another breech baby, right? Everything was going as smoothly as I hoped. I got into MGP, despite me thinking I would not be eligible. At 25 weeks, I was so happy, as the baby was head down. At 27 weeks, something changed; the movements felt different and scarily familiar. 28 weeks, it was confirmed that the baby was breech. Not again! I could not believe it. For 9 weeks, I tried everything possible to turn her around. All of the spinning babies' techniques, handstands in the pool, acupuncture and moxibustion, chiropractic, homeopathy, hypnosis, and more. I even asked about breech VBAC, but the hospital would not have supported it. I felt like I should have a degree in what tricks should turn a baby around. The time was approaching for when I could attempt an ECV. I kept seeing stories of this amazing doctor (practically the breech baby whisperer) turning all these babies and supporting breech birth for those he could not turn. He was in Sydney, and I was on the Gold Coast. It would be mad for me to try and go see him, right?

Well, I made a phone call to the Royal Hospital for Women and spoke with Dr. Bisits, and he agreed to see me. So, 37 weeks pregnant with my toddler in tow, we flew to Sydney to see him for an ECV. The procedure took barely minutes and was no more than slightly uncomfortable. It was a completely opposite experience to the attempt with my son. He did it! She turned! I finally had a baby head down. Four weeks later, at 40w + 8d, I had my empowering VBAC. I did require an episiotomy, due to significant bradycardia, although I was respectfully asked for consent, and I healed well. That VBAC high though, nothing compares. I rode that for at least 18 months.

2VBAC, May 2021 – Now, after having two previous breech babies, I had a one in three chance of having another.

I was lucky enough to have the same midwife, through the birth centre that I had for my daughter's birth. When I spoke with her, I said straight away, "What happens if this baby is breech?" She said that she would support me in a breech VBAC should it come to it.

Right from the 12-week scan, this baby was showing head up. My husband and I laughed at the ridiculousness of it. My 20-week scan came, and baby was still head up. At 28 weeks, baby was confirmed to be breech. This time, I focused my energy on spinning babies' exercises and chiropractic with Webster technique, trying to retrace the steps that I truly felt helped turn my daughter. I didn't want to be doing absolutely everything like last pregnancy, as trying to turn a breech baby can be time consuming.

Due to COVID, I was keeping a close eye on the interstate border, as I was starting to think I would need to go to Sydney again.

At 34 weeks, I contacted Dr. Bisits to request an ECV with him again. He happily accepted my request.

36w+6d, I flew to Sydney to see Dr. Bisits. The ECV was, again, a success. I stayed in Sydney until 37w+1d, and had a scan to confirm the position.

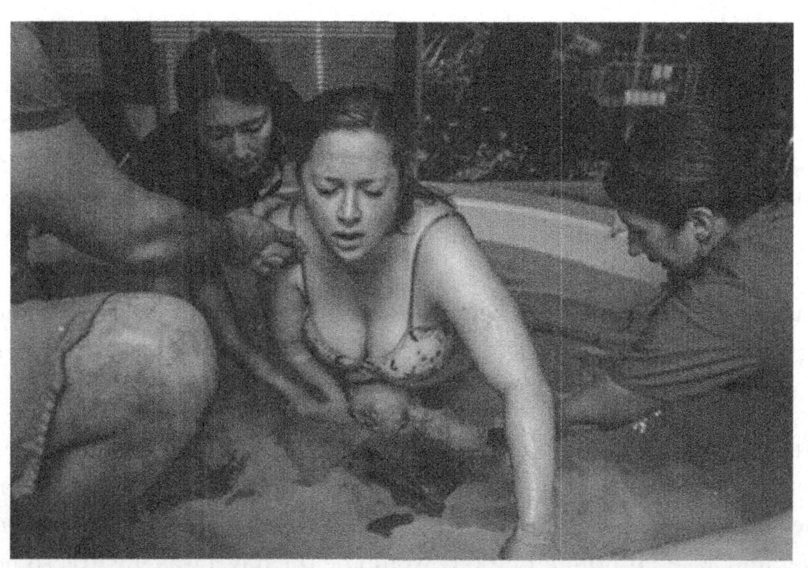

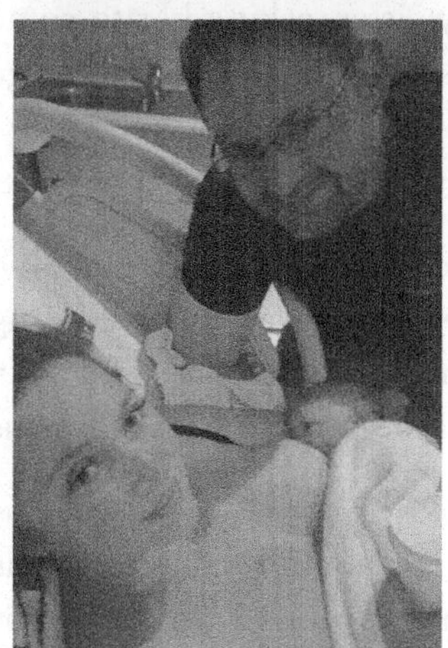

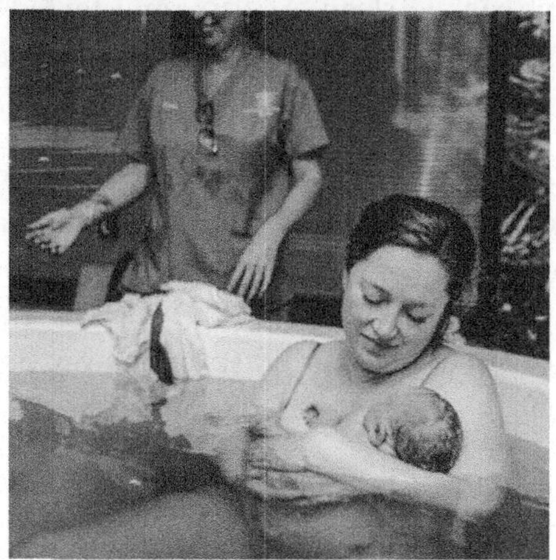

Siobhan Burrell, Queensland, Australia

The baby was still head down. I then flew home. Before leaving, I asked Dr. Bisits if he had come across many women who had had three consecutive breech babies in a row, and he said, "No, that is very much the trifecta!" I am so grateful to this man. All obstetricians should be like him.

I had had increasing Braxton Hicks contractions from approximately 35 weeks. At 39+5, I woke overnight with strong period pains, but they did not turn into anything, so I went back to sleep. The next morning, I had my midwife appointment. This was the first appointment since my return from Sydney. I was nervous that they would tell me that my baby had turned back to breech. I mentioned the period pains, but I brushed them off, as I had been having some mild period pains in the weeks leading up to that day. I expected to be pregnant for another week or so, despite jokingly saying, "Today would be good."

39+6, I woke at 1:30am to mild contractions. I began timing them. They were approximately 10 minutes apart. I just lay in bed, dozing between the contractions and timing them. Around 2:30 am, my husband rolled over and asked if I thought today would be the day. I was unsure, so he went back to sleep. At 3:30 am, I texted my sister, asking her to come over, hoping that she might get it. I said in the text that I would call if the contractions picked up anymore.

At 4 am, I realised I was not going back to sleep, and I decided to get up and have a cup of tea and some yogurt. I also put on my TENS machine. Not long after getting up, my daughter came out to see what I was doing. I took her back to bed, she asked to have a breastfeed, I let her latch, but I needed to take her off straight away, as it intensified the contractions too much.

At 4:30 am, I messaged my midwife to tell her about the contractions, as I was not sure about calling so early in the morning. I also called my sister to ask her to come over. She was a little dazed, and the conversation ended with her saying for me to let her know when to come over, to which I agreed. My eldest then woke. I then asked my husband to wake up. I had said to my sister that I would wait 20 min and see how I was going. At 4:55 am, I messaged my sister and told her she needed to come now.

At 5 am, I called my midwife to tell her my contractions were coming every 3 minutes and lasting a minute. She said she would meet us at the birth centre. I also called my birth photographer; she was so lovely and calming. We were getting ready, and my children just wanted to be near me. I hoped my sister would not be much longer. My husband called to check where she was, and she was only a few minutes away. My sister arrived at 5:25am, and we got straight into the car. My daughter was upset seeing me going through contractions, and my son wanted to come with us, and then he wanted to tell me something before we left. I told him I loved him, but I could not stay for a chat.

We arrived at the hospital at 6 am. My husband had planned to drop me off at the front. He pulled up and got the bag out of the car. I went to try and get out of the car, and another contraction came. I quickly got back in the car. A lady on her way into the hospital for work heard me and got me a wheelchair (much to my dislike, only because I didn't want to be in a chair). She was lovely. I didn't want my husband to leave me to park the car. The lady said she would wait with me. She started to take me towards the entrance, and my husband came running. We quickly made our way to the birth centre. Thankfully, my midwife met us as we arrived, and just as we were about to make our way to the birth suite, my birth photographer also arrived. My husband wheeled me into the room and parked me right in front of the bath.

I sat while I waited for my midwife to finish preparing for us and for the current contraction to pass. My midwife started preparing a mat and a birth ball for me. I knew all I wanted was to be in the water, and I asked if I could get in. She started running the water straight away.

My midwife said, "Siobhan, I will have to check if that baby is still head down" I had a laugh and agreed. I then got up onto the bed, where they checked my baby's heart rate and position. When my midwife palpated the position of the head, it was so painful because the baby was low, and it caused an immediate contraction. I rolled over and clung to the wall. I then went over to the bath and was wondering if I could get into the water. My midwife was typing something, so I just hopped in. She turned and was a little worried as the water was not warm enough for the baby, as the bath had not finished filling (whoops).

At first, I was resting in a seated position, but my midwife asked me to check and see if I could feel the baby's head. After the next contraction, I felt inside, and I could feel the bulging bag of waters and said that they were still intact. I needed to find a new position. I moved around until I found that on my knees was the most comfortable. The contractions were so strong and coming right on top of each other, with no breaks in between. I said to my midwife that I just need a little break. I soon asked for the gas and air, as I felt I was not coping with the continual contractions. The gas gave a little relief.

Another contraction came, and I felt a pop. I knew my waters had broken. It was not long, and I could feel that my body wanted to push, so I allowed it to. I naturally began panting, and I tried to slow it down. The pushing was strong, although I wanted to go slowly. Then, after about the second push, I could feel baby was almost out, but once the contraction finished, he slipped back upwards. In my mind, I was thinking, "Nooo! Don't go back up!" On the next push, my baby's head was born. My midwife said to reach and touch his head, I did, and I still remember the gentle swishing of his hair in my hand. I then felt his head turn between my legs as he rotated. It felt like a long time until the next contraction came to birth his body, but it came. At 6:52am, my baby was born. I felt frozen to reach through to receive him. My student midwife was behind and guided him to come through to the front for me to bring him to the surface. As he was rising, my midwife said, "The cord is too tight!" It was wrapped around his neck. I quickly unravelled it and pulled him to my chest and collapsed to the side of the pool. We caught our breath, and someone told me to check if the baby was a boy or a girl. I lifted him up and checked.

I had a giggle and said to my husband that he would have to pick a name now (he could not settle on a boy's name at all). Soon, my midwife advised me that I would need to come out of the pool so that the placenta could be born. I made my way out and over to the bed. The placenta was born physiologically about 20 minutes after. No management was required. The afterpains kept coming, and they were stronger than I recall after my first VBAC. They eventually eased off, and I showered. I had a small second-degree tear (a five-minute second stage probably didn't help that). We were discharged 4 hours after birth, less than 5 hours after arriving at the birth centre.

Had he not turned cephalic spontaneously or by ECV, I would have gone forward with a breech VBAC. My husband and my midwife would have supported me. This was so healing to know that no matter what way my baby was presenting, I would not feel pressured to have another caesarean from the people who meant the most. After such a crazy journey with my children, I almost wish I had a breech birth, but sadly, I don't think my final birthing experience would have been as calm (by external influences, like the obstetrics team).

It was the perfect way to end the birthing phase of my life with no VEs, no cannula, no CTG, and no intervention. As far as hospital births go, it was as close to home birth as you can get with only people known to me in the room, and I was treated with complete support and respect.

I have no uterine anomalies that would make breech babies more likely. I will never know why my babies all sat breech, but I now feel like it was all for a reason. Due to my experiences with my children, I have been inspired to now support other women through their journeys. After the birth of my daughter, my first VBAC, I commenced working towards one day becoming a midwife. I feel like I needed to have this experience. I needed to be able to completely accept breech birth for myself so that I will one day be able to effectively support other women with babies that also present breech.

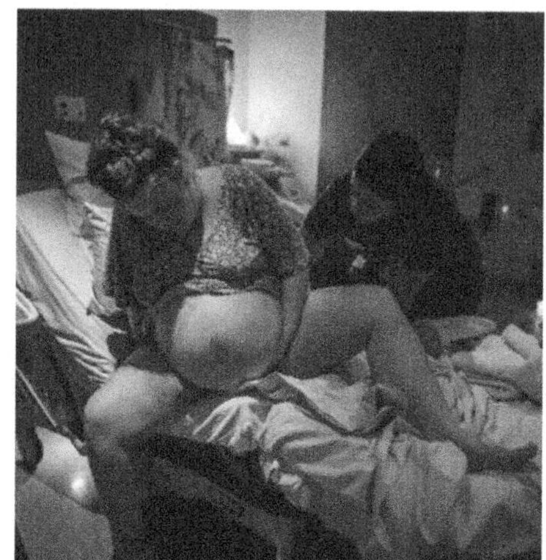

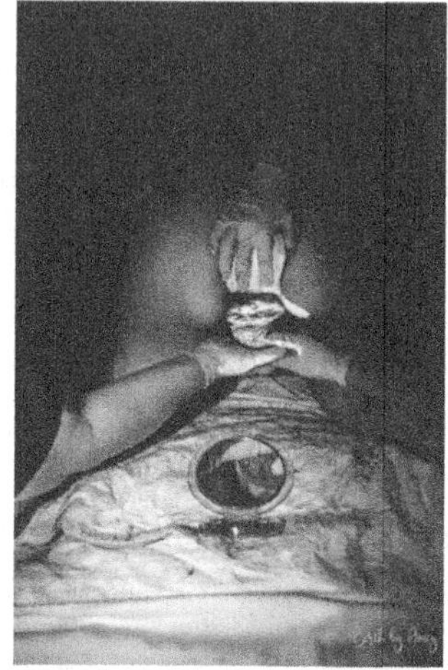

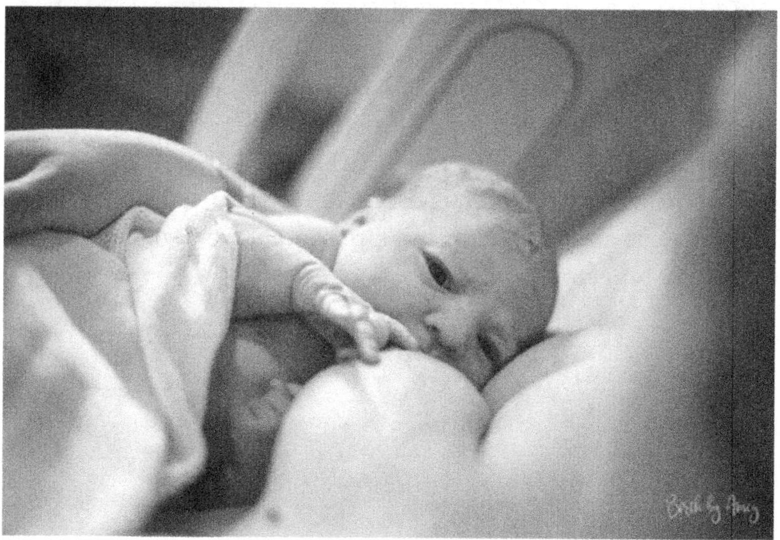

Danielle Chorley, ACT, Australia

Danielle –VBAC after 3 Caesareans (VBA3C)

There are 3 births before this one!

Baby 1, 2009, born at 40+10. Spontaneous labour. 5 cm when presenting to hospital. Didn't believe I was in labour, as I seemed to be not in much pain. Eventual epidural (unsuccessful). 12 hrs labour at hospital. Birth on back. No tears. Weight of 4.1kg.

Baby 2, 2011, born at 42+2. Spontaneous labour. Fast labour. Emergency c-section at 10 cms, as baby's heartbeat was lost. 15 minutes from red button call to baby out. Baby perfect scores. Weight of 5kg. PND and PTSD afterward.

Baby 3, 2018. Gravidarum hyperemesis throughout pregnancy until birth. Planned VBAC. Eventual elective section at 40+5 due to GH and pneumonia. Gentle C-section. Weight of 3.6kg. Baby fine.

There was also a missed miscarriage at 14 weeks between babies 2 and 3. D&C performed at my request in hospital.

I am currently in ACT, Australia, but as a military family, we move a lot. My first 2 babies were born in Queensland, D&C in NSW, and the last two births were in Canberra.

Birth Story of Artemis Willa – VBA2C

Born: 17/3/2020

Weight: 4.07kg

CW: Meconium, previous c-sections, general obstetric hijinks

Be forewarned, it's a long one. I'm going right back to my booking in appointment for context. I alternated care between the hospital and my GP (who is so amazing and woman-centred that I wished she'd been an OB).

16-week apt: Booking in appointment at the local public hospital. The midwife asked if I was planning another c-section (I have had 1 vaginal, 1 emerge section, and 1 elect section). I told her, "No, I will be having a

VBAC." The midwife smiled, said, "Wonderful," and told me she was excited for me. We did all the standard paperwork, etc. I told her to calculate my due date from ovulation, not last period (I have a long cycle and have tracked ovulation for a while). This is vital here; it gave me an extra week wiggle room as far as the OBs were concerned. This gave me an official due date of March 8th. It would have been March 1st by LMP.

20-week apt (after scan): The baby was all good and sizing well. The registrar OB was supportive of my desire for a VBA2C. She went through the pros and cons of both and made a note that I had been well counselled. She did ask if I would do another scan to check size at 28 weeks. I refused. She conceded and made a note to check with the head OB (he was down with it all).

28-week apt: Standard midwife apt. Nothing at all mentioned about c-section. They made sure I knew the signs of labour and what to do if I felt I needed assistance, etc.

34-week apt: A different registrar OB. She went over the pros and cons again of both options. She did, however, go and get one of the three head OBS for a chat. This man, a talented surgeon, who is a great doctor (especially for women who have fertility issues) absolutely did not support my VBA2C. We had a good 20-minute battle, which ended in him conceding and asking if I agreed to see him again in a few weeks. He also said he would be sending me to the other public hospital, as the one I was at couldn't support me through a VBA2C. I told him to do what he thought best. I then continued to ignore the booking in calls from the other hospital. (Please note I work for the public hospital I planned to birth in; I knew their rules and regs inside and out.)

38-week apt: Cancelled and rescheduled for 10 days later. I couldn't be bothered to fight OB again, and just went to my GP for a wellness check.

39+3-week apt: The not-supportive OB goes over all his previous points. I do not budge except to tell him I'm happy for CTG monitoring every second day, and for a growth scan. I was happy to do this anyway for my peace of mind but warned him that no matter how big they said the baby was, that information was going to bother him more than me.

40-week scan: Baby well, prediction of 5.7kg

40-week apt: A brisk 5-min check from not-happy OB, and a small word of encouragement from two separate midwives. Apparently, this saga was being followed with interest.

40+5-week CTG scan: Ambushed by head of surgery, the other head OB, a registrar OB, and midwife. They wanted to go over in writing what the plan was. I told them I will see how it all goes and how it feels on the day. They wanted to book a just-in-case section. I said, no. Cannula. No. I told them these things weren't set in stone, and I was all for seeing what happened. The head of surgery and OB were sceptical (both male), and the registrar and midwife supportive (both female).

Now, the birth bit:

I had irritable uterus from about 25 weeks with this baby. It was a pain in the arse.

I went into prodromal labour at about 40+5 (41+5 by LMP). On and off. Enough to be annoying but nothing further.

On Thursday 12th of March, I lost my plug. Just the plug (no blood) in one beautiful clump. Mild cramping continued for days. On Sunday the 15th, I started having a show. Light bleeding with cramps, only enough to wipe when using the toilet.

On Monday the 16th, contractions started to gain traction but were coming in various patterns. My mum came and collected my two oldest sons (10 and 8) and took them back to her house. Eventually, the contractions started to come more frequently and gain in strength. They were lasting for 40 seconds and coming every 2 mins roughly, but I could still kind of talk through them. We phoned my doula for advice. She got me to lean off the sofa onto my head (held by my husband) to use gravity to move the baby out of the pelvis a bit. She theorized all this prodromal labour was the baby getting into good position, and maybe she just needed a little room. I held it for 15 seconds and down. Within 20 minutes, the contractions were really there, and I was vocalising through them.

I called Mum back with the boys (to come and look after the toddler), and for our doula to come over.

My timings get fuzzy here, so they are all estimates.

The doula arrived at 11 to 11:30. My hubby swapped out with her so he could get the bags together. I started to need counter pressure, and my vocalisation increased. The TENS was turned up and heat packs added.

At about 1 to 1:30 am, I asked to be taken to the hospital; the pain was getting more than I could handle at home and I was being awfully noisy. Off we went.

I had a mini breakdown in the car, worried for mine and my baby's safety. I was scared I'd made the wrong decision. The hubby gave me a pep talk and held my hand. Contractions slowed a little bit. There was a huge, beautiful moon to look at, though.

We arrived at hospital, and it took about 15 mins to get up to birth suite, as the contractions came back hard and fast. I had to stop and lean into my husband every 10 metres. I was offered a wheelchair by nurse in ED but couldn't think of anything worse at that moment. We made it to the birth suite and were met by one of my beautiful midwives. We were taken straight to a suite with a bath and a shower. I was labouring while leaning on the bed when the duty OB came in. He wanted to discuss cannula. I had 3 contractions while this happened. He stopped each time and waited for me. I told him that I appreciate his expertise, but that at the moment I am fine, and will absolutely let him know if I need him, and he left. I did not see an OB again until the wellness check for baby.

I told the midwife that I was happy to wear the wireless monitor for 20 mins for their peace of mind but would not keep it on. All good. I stripped and got into the shower with the monitor on. My student midwife arrived here at some point. The other midwife essentially left us to it. My student midwife did all the Doppler monitoring (I only noticed her doing it once, but she did it every 20 mins or so).

I ripped off the monitors eventually because they were annoying me and stayed in that sweet shower for about 2 hrs. At about 4 am, I asked for an internal (my first and only), as I wanted to know how far I was in relation to my pain. I jumped on the bed and found out that I was a stretchy 6 cms. I was a little defeated, honestly, but my husband, doula, and midwives roused me and got me back in the shower.

About an hour later (5 am), I was begging for pain relief during contractions. I didn't think I could keep going. My team reminded me I didn't want pain relief if I could avoid it. They said it was most likely too late for morphine and even an epi. My beautiful student midwife took a leap of faith and offered gas. I had strictly said not to offer it to me, as I hated it during my first birth, but I jumped on it like nothing before.

I'm so glad she did. I got up on all fours over the back of the bed and sucked on that amazing gas. As you can imagine, it went quite hazy at this point, and time lost all meaning. Once I had the knack of it, my contractions were mostly painless, except at their peak. My midwife and doula noted the musty smell that often occurs when women are near full dilation. My husband stayed by my side and held me when needed. There was music, snacks, and laughter. I apologised in advance if I pooped on anyone. My doula stood on the bed and used a scarf to relieve by back pain and was the recipient of a bag of exploding waters all down her legs.

There was meconium in the water, but as far as I knew, no one was concerned. Eventually, my vocalisations turned into mooing grunts. At about 6 am, I started to push. I followed my body and was only coached at one point to stop pushing and pant, so as not to tear. My student midwife assisted the head midwife in protecting my perineum as requested. There was a slight ring of fire and, at 6:25 am, out sprang baby Artemis, covered in vernix and poo.

Her cord was quite short. She was passed up between my legs and placed on my belly while we waited for white. The afterpains were insane, so I sucked on the gas while we waited for the placenta. Dad cut her cord once white.

I had a small 1 cm tear, not requiring stitches, and for the first time in four births, I was the first person to hold my baby. I did not let her go for 2 hrs. She had a feed, and when I was ready, my doula helped me shower while Daddy oversaw her wellness checks.

I was ecstatic. We were all so chilled. Our doula went and got us breakfast, and we basked in our new baby glow. The head of surgery visited and apologised for not believing in me and my instinct that she would not be 5.7 kg. He would like to debrief with me further at some point. I ran into not-happy OB in the hall on our way out, and he did not make eye contact.

Anyway, I warned you it was long. You can do this, ladies. You got this. Back yourself and find a team who will back you too. It's a long game, but worth it.

Naomi – VBAC with an Inverted T Scar

Water birth after inverted-T-incision caesarean

My VBAC story starts with my first birth. My first pregnancy was a planned and exciting pregnancy, but overall uneventful. I planned on a homebirth and was excited when my contractions started at 40 weeks, 5 days. The contractions came hard and fast but then eased off a few hours later. I slept in between the irregular contractions, and the next morning, they started strengthening up again, so I got into the birth pool. A while later, I noticed something in the bottom of the pool and thought it might be some bloody show. I felt inside my vagina and felt something quite hard, like a closed cervix, which disappointed me, as I had hoped all my contractions overnight might have started opening it.

As I pulled my fingers out, I realized it looked more like meconium in the pool. I checked again and immediately burst into tears, saying, "I don't want a caesarean." What I thought was a cervix was a heel. What I was feeling was an entire little foot sitting at the introitus of my vagina. I called my midwives to attend and when they arrived, they confirmed that it was a footling breech, and I was 6 cm dilated.

As they were confident and trained in birthing breech babies, we decided to stay at home and see if my labour would continue to progress. Four hours later, my midwife did another vaginal examination. There was no change, and I was beginning to get tired from the long night/day of contractions. We made the decision to transfer to hospital, a 2 ½ hour drive away. When my midwife consulted with the obstetrician on call, he ordered a helicopter and I transferred to the hospital. On my arrival to the hospital, the obstetrician on call checked me and stated that I was fully dilated with a footling breech. He recommended a caesarean section, but as there was no fetal distress, we decided to wait for my partner to arrive, since he had to drive down.

While I waited, I pushed and pushed, despite not having an overwhelming urge to do so. The tiny foot slowly began to protrude further out my introitus. I was so determined to avoid a caesarean section.

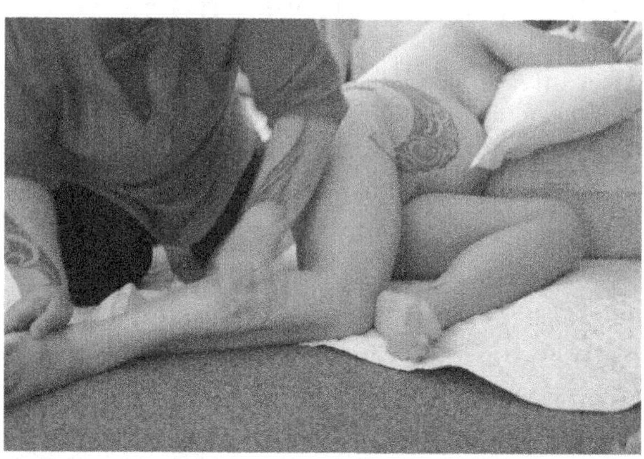

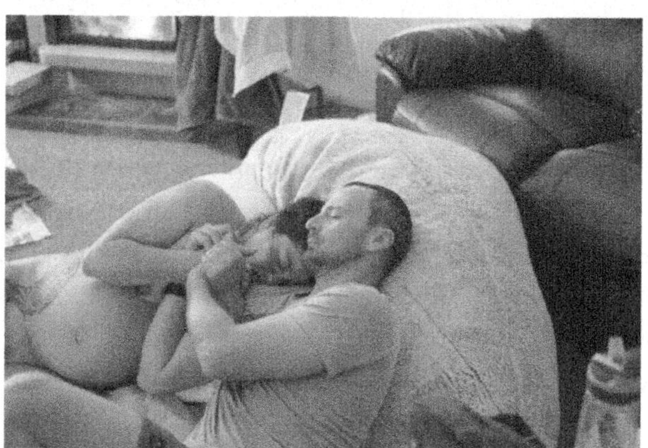

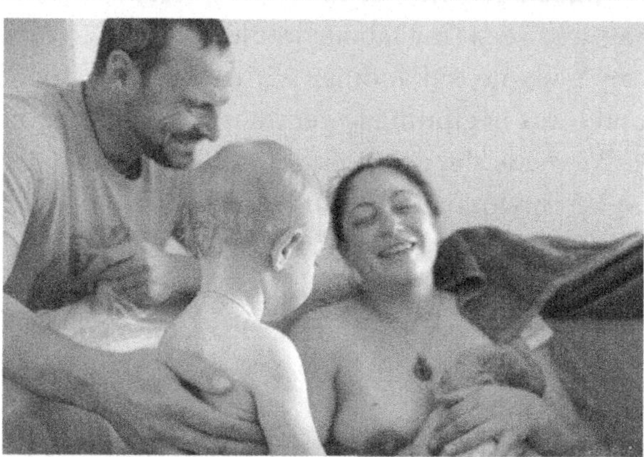

Naomi Waldron, Cable Bay, New Zealand

When my partner arrived, the obstetrician assessed me again. There was no descent, the foot protruding was simply the leg extending, but the baby was not coming. So, the decision was made that we proceed for a caesarean section.

The next morning, the obstetrician came to see me and explained it was a difficult surgery. The baby's head was entrapped under my ribs and was unable to be extracted, even with the extension of the transverse incision. He then made an incision 8 cm vertically to form an inverted T. It was still difficult to birth the baby, so forceps were needed. The baby came out and needed to be resuscitated but was able to come and meet me within 10 minutes. I cried when I heard about the complications of my surgery, as I knew that the recommendation was for all future births to be elective caesareans.

The healing, both mentally and physically, was hard, but I made an effort to not push myself physically and allow myself to feel all the raw emotions and grieve my lost homebirth that I had envisioned.

I fell pregnant again when my son was 9 months old. Physically, I had an easy pregnancy. I was able to continue my boxing classes until I stopped work at 8-months pregnant. My scar stretched and I felt nothing. I wouldn't have known I had a scar, apart from the fact I could see it. The only pregnancy symptom I had was intense nipple pain when breastfeeding, but I was determined to continue feeding, as my son was still so young.

Emotionally, it was a hard pregnancy. At 22 weeks, I had a scan that showed my placenta was over the vertical part of my scar. As I tried to prepare mentally for my birth, there was also the consideration that I may have a morbidly adhered placenta and I risked hemorrhaging and a hysterectomy.

I was still determined to try for a vaginal birth, as I knew I would always regret it if I didn't try. I did a lot of research into placenta accreta and uterine rupture. I also live 2 ½ hours away from a hospital with obstetric services, so I had to consider how I would transfer in labour.

A scan at 36 weeks showed that the placenta was still over the vertical part of my scar but had moved and did not look to be an accreta. We decided to book accommodation that was 10 minutes away from the hospital and I would stay there from 39 weeks to await labour.

At 39 weeks, I was settling into the house we had rented for a couple of weeks, and I was breastfeeding my son to sleep when I felt my contractions start. They felt intense and were coming about 4 mins apart. I called my midwife to let her know, as she was 2 ½ drive away and she came. She was happy to support me to birth at the rental house, knowing we were less than 10 minutes away from the hospital if we needed it.

After a couple of hours, the contractions eased off a bit and I felt a bit disheartened that I had called for a false alarm. At 3 am, my waters broke and although I was tired, I felt excited that something was finally happening. I thought I would have a few strong contractions and then have a baby. It took 30 minutes for my contractions to start again, and although they were more intense, they remained irregular. I moved around and got into the birth pool.

At 6 am, I was starting to get really tired, and I didn't feel like I had made much progress, as it didn't feel like the baby had descended. I asked for a vaginal exam and my midwife said I was 4 cm, and the head was still high. I felt disappointed, as I had been contracting on and off for the whole night. As the fetal heart rate was normal and I was tired but coping, I was determined to carry on. I asked for sacral pressure during contractions. I was so aware of my body, my baby, and my scar, but my scar never worried me, as it never felt uncomfortable. I knew I needed my hips to open more to help the baby descend, so I asked the two midwives to push on my hips and lower back. I kept asking them to push harder, knowing their arms were aching but also knowing that this was what my body needed. I felt it working, I felt the baby move lower and yet, I didn't have an urge to push, and I was rapidly running out of energy. Just before 10 am, I asked my midwife to do another vaginal examination and push my cervix out of the way if there was just a little bit. As she checked me, I gave a little push and felt the last bit of cervix disappear. Finally, I was fully dilated. I got back into the pool and waited for contractions so I could push my baby out. The head was still quite high, as I didn't have a strong urge to push, but as I was so tired, I just wanted the labour to be over so I pushed as hard as I could.

It was amazing to feel that it was working, and I was in control of it. With each push, I felt the baby move lower. My contractions eased off to 5 to 6 minutes apart, so I rested in between and then pushed. I felt my baby's head as it was crowning and slowly let it stretch me. After the head was born, I waited impatiently for the next contraction. With the next contraction, I pushed and reached down to pick my baby up, but he was not coming. In a tired voice, I said, "help me." My midwife reached down and helped his body out. His hand was by his face, which explained why I had irregular contractions, as his head was acynclitic, as evidenced by the molding on one side of his head.

At 11:05am, my partner reached into the water and placed our baby on my chest. I did it.

The cord continued to pulse for about 15 minutes, then the placenta separated and came away easily by itself with minimal blood loss.

This is the birth I had been dreaming of and hoping for.

Being surrounded by support people that believed in me and supported me throughout my labour made me able to cope with it. The skills of the midwives to help the baby move lower and the willingness to support me, even though I did not have continuous monitoring and was not in a hospital, are the things that prevented me from having a repeat caesarean.

I am so grateful that I had a choice, and I was able to make the informed choice that was right for me and achieve what I set out to. I wish all women had an option to choose the birth they wanted.

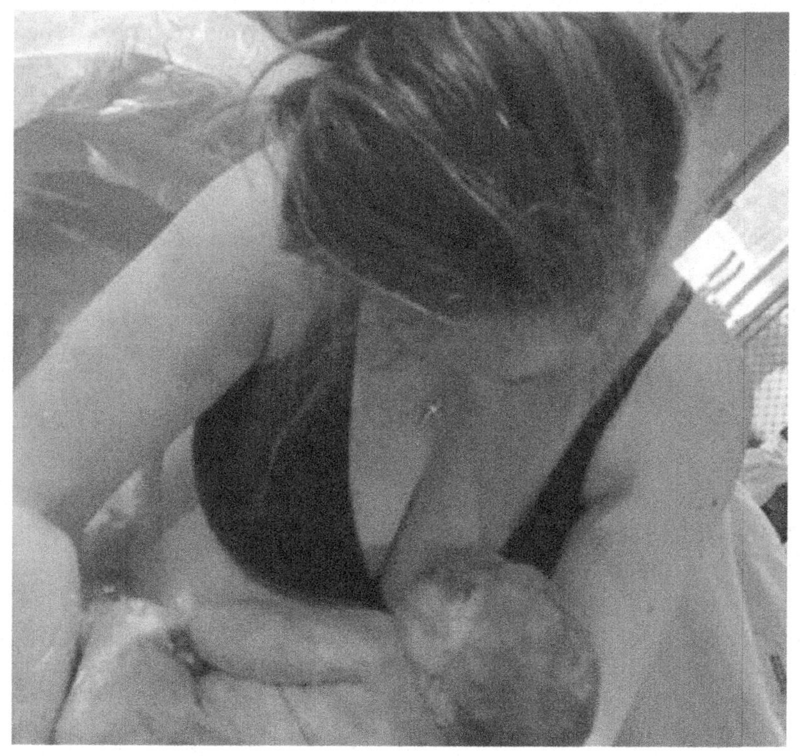

Emili Raguz, NSW, Australia

Emili – Homebirth after 2 Caesareans

My dream of giving birth the way I hoped for: natural, without any interventions and being in some sort of control and reaching that absolute bliss when the baby comes out was shattered when I got diagnosed with GD with my firstborn.

From that day, everything changed. Although my GD was diet-controlled and all went well, I couldn't go pass 40+6 weeks.

When the time came, I went to hospital to be induced. After 36 hours of labour, I had to have emergency c-section, failure to progress, and pushing for too long.

Being a first-time mum, I had no idea what went wrong and why my body failed me. My baby's safety was my top priority, so I felt like failure. I was emotional and upset, and cried through the whole process. My son was born 4.3 kg and I was relieved that all went well.

After two years, I fell pregnant again.

This time around, I didn't have GD but because of the previous c-section, I was told I'd need it again.

I can't remember how I came upon a VBAC meeting at Blacktown hospital where I was booked, as with previous pregnancy. Did my midwife mention it, or did I see their flyer? That first meeting was a huge eye-opener.

It was led by an amazing midwife called Sue. I learnt many things. I wrote down everything she said, and I was filled with hope that this time, I might have the birth I want. One thing she said I still remember: fight for it. You have to fight for your birth and don't let them win. I was so full of hope and optimism when I had next obstetric appointment and it all popped like a balloon when I said to OB that I want to have VBAC and he replied, "How would you feel if your baby dies because of you?"

I can't remember what I answered but I do remember that I rang my husband once in the car and couldn't stop crying. Every appointment I had, the OB used scare tactic to make me change my mind. Sue and other pregnant mamas were giving me strength, and we were each other beacon of hope.

At 40 weeks appointment, I was dilated 4 cm, I thought that surely this time, the baby will come early. Nope, nothing. At 41 weeks, the husband drove me to hospital. They broke my waters, and everything went fast forward, like in movies.

After 4 hours or so, it was time to push. Sue just finished her shift and popped in for moral support. I pushed and pushed but nothing happened. All this time, I was upright or kneeling. I got told to lay on my back, as they need to examine me. After that, I felt like it was an out-of-body experience. I wanted to get up, as I wasn't comfortable on my back. I got told that the baby needs to get out and I need to stay where I was. I did not want to lay on bed because it didn't feel right. I had two midwives holding my legs and pushing knees towards my stomach, and the other midwife was pushing on my stomach. Suddenly, there was a group of people all looking at my vagina, to my husband's annoyance, who was holding my arm, and Sue, the other. Another midwife was using a suction cap to pull the baby out, and after 12 years, I still remember the feeling and the noise it made. The suction cap didn't work so she had to use forceps, and I got told that they need to do episiotomy, as the baby had shoulder dystocia. All this time, I was told to push, push, push.

All I was thinking was that this can't be happening. It's all a bad dream. What the hell is going on?

To be honest, I was hoping that I died and for all the pain I was experiencing to be gone. I don't know how long it went for, but it felt like forever.

There was a lot of commotion and pressure, and all of sudden, they put my son on me. The first thing I thought was, "oh, my poor baby, what you have to go through to come out!"

He was 5.100kg and I couldn't believe it. His head was like a cone, but it went down afterwards. His shoulder was fine, and they checked his sugars via heel prick, and all was well.

I felt like a superwoman. I was over the moon that I finally got my VBAC.

He was the biggest baby at hospital, and he got lots of visits from midwives, as he was a star attraction.

After a few years, I fell pregnant again, and this time, I was booked in Windsor hospital. I think it's called St. John of God now.

I got diagnosed with GD, and because of my previous birth history, I got told that I cannot be induced, and if I don't go into labor by 40 weeks, I had to have a c-section.

I tried everything in books to induce the labour naturally. At one point, my husband bought me 5 kg of pineapples, as supposedly, that does the trick. I couldn't feel my lips for days, and still nothing happened. I felt let down by my body again and couldn't believe I'm, yet again, facing c-section. I signed the form for elective section, although there was nothing elective about it. I didn't want to have c-section but there were no other options. Before I sign the letter, OB said he had to examine me to see if my cervix was favourable.

It was only me and him, and I said I wanted midwife present. He said it will be quick and the midwives are busy, and he doesn't want to bother them with such an insignificant thing.

I should've said no, but I obliged.

It did not feel right and I hated myself.

He said, "Cervix is thick and the only way this baby will come out is by c-section."

When the day came, I was upset that, once again, my body failed me.

My son was born 4.5 kg and all was well.

After 5 years, I had a miscarriage. I was 4 weeks and didn't even realise I was pregnant.

Two years after that, I had another miscarriage. This time, I was 10 weeks and it happened at home.

I knew that there was nothing I can do besides letting my body overtake. I surrendered myself, and from this loss, I gained trust that my body knows what it's doing and what's natural. From that day, I look at my body different, with respect.

After 2 years, I fell pregnant again, and having two previous miscarriages and considering I was 41, I thought for sure that I will lose this baby as well.

So every time I would go to the toilet, I looked back, thinking there will be blood.

But there wasn't, and after 3 months, I thought, "Okay, time to go to go for hospital referral."

We moved to Central Coast then, and I booked in Gosford hospital.

It was 2020, and when COVID happened, restrictions started to begin, and hospital had policy that children are not allowed to come to appointments and to visit the baby. The tiny voice inside me said, "This is it. This is your chance. It's time."

On first booking, I told the midwife that I want to have a VBAC. She was positive that it could happen, but we need to consider my birth history and not to get my hopes up, in case I end up with another c-section.

All was going well. I decline a Glucose test, and instead, I finger-pricked myself every day to make sure my sugar levels were good. I did not want to be defined by GD again. I knew that I would have a big baby again, and I've done lots and lots of reading and research into shoulder dystocia, and what to do if it's present.

I've also started following all the inspirational midwives, especially Martina Gorner. That little light called "hope" was starting to shine a bit brighter.

On every appointment, they would talk about risk of scar ruptures and brain damage, and asked questions like:

-What will your husband say to your other kids if you die in labour?

-How would you feel, knowing that you could have normal, healthy baby, and instead, got one with brain damage. Do you realise how that would that change your family?

I said once that this is my last baby and I want to experience natural birth again, and the lady OB said, "Well, we can tie your tubes for you if you have a c-section."

I was gobsmacked. "Would they suck the stomach fat as well?" I was about to ask, but kept my mouth shut.

At 32 weeks, I got told point blank that hospital won't allow me to birth any other way except c-section unless I go into labour naturally. They couldn't induce me and there is no other way.

I was furious and I said to myself that this is the last time I set my foot here.

Every time after appointments, I would start having panic attacks, and after the last appointment the next day, as I was driving my kids to school, I had a bad one and I hated my kids seeing me like that, but I promised myself I will not birth at that hospital, and it's time I take my power back.

I talked to my husband about hiring a private midwife, and everything was going okay, until I mentioned I want to have a water birth. At that point, it clicked for him what it actually means not to hire a midwife for a hospital birth but for homebirth.

Hahaha! The look on his face was priceless.

I got recommendations for a great midwife, Karyn, and I emailed her. Because I was already late in pregnancy, I was crossing my fingers and toes. She was booked for the rest of the year, except September, when I was due.

Meant to be.

What is there to say about Karyn? How can I describe her and not feel endless gratitude and love for her? I never met such a caring and calm midwife. I was in excellent hands. We came to an agreement that if I don't go into labour by 40+ weeks, we would try and see if hospital would at least break my waters. Then came the ultrasound, which confirmed that the baby was big.

I will never forget when she said that there is a possibility that if the baby comes after 40+ weeks, it might be 6 or more kilos, going by ultrasound measurements. At that point, my vagina was silently screaming.

Giving that all my boys were 41 weeks, I was expecting the same with this baby.

At 36 weeks, I bought pram and washed all my baby clothes.

At 36+5 days, I got the baby capsule installed. I drove home, then patted the belly and said, "Okay, baby, all is set. You can come out now" and to myself, thinking, "Yeah, right. There is at least another month or so."

At 2:20 am on my first day of 37 weeks, I felt like I was wetting myself. I got up and my water broke.

How to describe that feeling?

Elation! Pure elation.

I could not believe it.

My husband was in Sydney, so I rang him to come straight away.

My oldest son got up and started to clear the room for the birth pool, bless him. He also started writing down contraction times. Karyn was on her way. My other two boys were sleeping. Once Karyn came, her and my husband set up the pool, and I was in.

It felt so peaceful and calm, and I never once asked if she has anything for pain relief.

I wanted to experience birth as it should be before society told us that that's not the way. Why suffer when there is pain relief?

To each their own and whatever every woman wants and needs, it should be accommodated.

Everything was going good. My baby and my heartbeat were fine, and at one point, I wanted to experience what I saw other women do; reach down and feel how far the baby's head was. So, I did, and to my surprise, I touched the baby's head. It was surreal. I was supposed to push but I was stalling. Why?

Because, in my head, there were scenes playing from my second birth. I was suddenly scared that something will go wrong and that my baby will die.

Yes, scare tactics from obstetrician were working. My baby's head is so close and all I'm thinking is, "My baby will die. What have I done?"

There was also the second midwife, Heidi, and she was simply amazing as well. She used acupuncture to turn the baby and to ease my contraction pain, and she was a wonderful support.

After mustering the courage to push with each surge and to have trust in my body, my baby's head was starting to rotate but it kept coming out, then in again. With an almighty roar, my baby was pushed out. I went down to reach for her and placed her on my chest. Yes, it was a she, I found out after few minutes. She was precious, all covered in vernix and quiet.

I was worried, as she didn't make a sound. She was taking it all in. We had to get out of water, as it was getting cold and it was time to get the placenta out.

I had to have a shot for the placenta to be released and didn't need any stitches. I had a small tear and that's it.

She was 4.9kg, and thank Heavens she came early. I don't think I would have done it if she was 6kg!

With her arrival, my circle of birth is closed and thanks to her, healed.

At the end, I got what I always wanted: an undisturbed and calm birth.

If I can have my time again, I would tell my younger self to hire a private midwife and a doula, if possible, and birth at home, not to listen to voices of doubt, and to trust her body first and foremost.

Despite everything I experienced, I am grateful for all my births, and for those wonderful midwives' who work tirelessly, give their best, and do their job with care and respect for women.

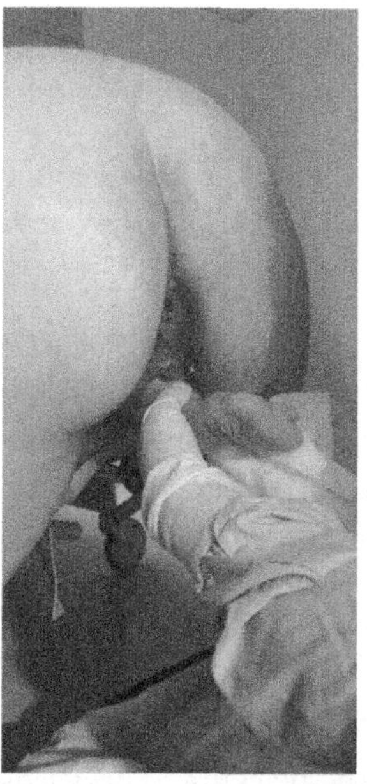

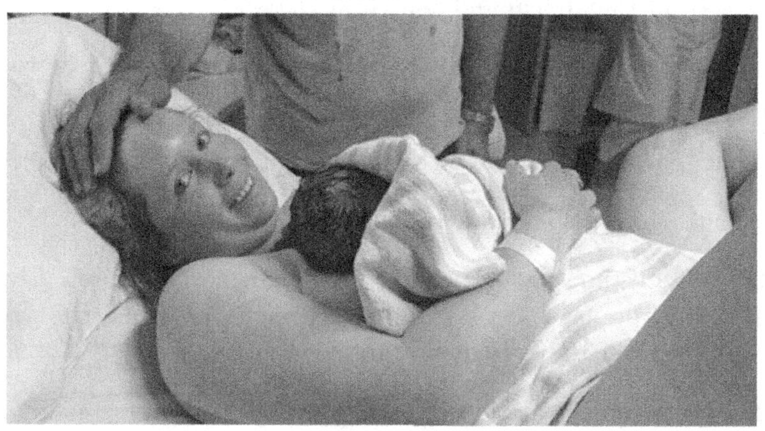

Hayley Karamian

Hayley – Breech VBAC

I think I probably started planning a home birth for my second baby before I was out of theatre after my first baby was cut out of me [for breech presentation]. I can remember debriefing with my birth centre midwives and being told that I couldn't birth at the birth centre now, and so I certainly couldn't have a home birth through the hospital either.

Arthur and I decided that we would start talking about another baby when Caleb was 2 years old, as 2 seemed to be the magic number to wait between pregnancies for those keen for a VBAC.

Most of my pregnancy was dominated by COVID-19, lockdown, and all that ensued from that. I felt so relieved to have secured Rachele (privately practicing midwife) in February, because shortly after that, homebirth had become a popular choice suddenly, and midwives became busier than ever.

My pregnancy was uneventful, just like my first. Because I was running after a 2-year-old, I didn't have time to fuss about every little symptom. I didn't feel any nausea at all and felt normal hunger. I was definitely exhausted, but this time, I knew there was no helping it, so I just kept going and didn't have any days off to rest.

Rachele was always confident in a head-down position, but Arthur and I still decided to go for the ultrasound at 36 weeks. Rachele just wrote a generic referral and the technician seemed somewhat bemused when I said that I was only there to determine the baby's position, even though nobody thought he was breech, but immediately upon putting down the wand, she identified his head right below my ribs. This was such a huge shock and an emotional time for me, as I saw my chances of a home birth and even a natural birth unravelling. It brought up all of the pain of my first son's surprise breech caesarean, terrible recovery, and emotional trauma. I was still hopeful, as the baby was measuring at a good size, only one week ahead, and I had no other complications besides being VBAC.

I messaged Rachele immediately, and we enacted our plan that we had ready, and went to see Dr. Smith, the breech OB at the Hospital, for the following Monday, at exactly 37 weeks. Seeing as I had gone to so much trouble to avoid hospitals and doctors, and had read so many horror stories about obstetricians, I was nervous when I went in. Rachele met me there, and we sat and waited, all masked up.

I told him the story of my first birth, an undiagnosed breech. He was sympathetic and said that it was not the first time that he had heard a story like mine, and that had I been at Westmead then, I would have been given other options if I wanted to continue to birth naturally. Undiagnosed breech does happen, and people do make mistakes like that all the time. We talked about the option to go for an ECV and what that involved. I could just have the baby breech in the hospital and not worry about an ECV, but he didn't recommend a breech home birth. I said that I was not worried about giving birth to a breech baby, but I didn't want to give birth in a hospital, because I didn't feel safe there. He seemed genuinely sad for me that I felt this way and he assured me that whatever happened, caesarean or natural birth, myself and my baby would be alright. He sounded so sincere that I felt bad for giving him such a hard time and started to relax. I could tell that he was supposed to outline caesarean as an option, but when I said that I knew about caesareans and didn't want to talk about that option, he said, "Yes, I sense that," moved right on, and didn't mention it again. He assured me that VBAC was no issue for breech, and I had as much chance as a FTM to have a normal delivery, so about 70% at that hospital, down from 80% if the baby's was head down. Otherwise, the baby was not looking too big from the ultrasound measurements and judging by my previous labour, I was a good candidate.

The ECV was not successful, but everyone was professional and kind to me. They monitored the baby for about 30 minutes, then put in a cannula and gave me medication to relax my muscles. Dr. Smith had a good go, using the ultrasound to check the baby's position as they went. It felt like getting a bad Chinese burn on my stomach and was definitely a lot harder to tolerate than I thought.

At 39+5 weeks, I found myself lying awake at 1:45 am, listening to my toddler falling back to sleep after a brief wakeup. Arthur had got up to get him a bottle and was in our bedroom. I had long since moved to the spare room, which would become the baby's room, as I was having so much trouble sleeping. It didn't help much. I got up to go to the toilet, as was my habit as soon as I woke up these days but was surprised to find I didn't need to wee. This was unusual for me at this point, but it had happened a few days ago when I was at work too. I went back to bed, and all of a sudden, I felt a slight cramp, and before I had time to wonder if this might be a contraction, I felt my waters break and literally flood my bed. Of course, my first thought was wanting to save the mattress, so I jumped up immediately and scrambled around for a pad. I tried to put a pad between my legs, but this did nothing; the waters were pouring out of me right through to the floor. I scrambled around for the big lady nappies, and this finally stemmed the flow. I stripped the bed and was relieved to see that the mattress was dry and even more relieved that the waters were clear of meconium.

I went in to tell Arthur, and he got up straight away and started packing, ready to go. I had no contractions yet and was in no hurry to leave and told him so. I texted Rachele to let her know, and then hung out in the bathroom for a bit and had a poo. Rachele didn't respond, so Arthur said I should call to let her know. I did and she was excited. I immediately asked if I could stay home and go back to sleep. She said that that was fine. Have a rest and let her know if things changed. I put fresh sheets on the bed and told Arthur to go back to bed (which he didn't do). I was just about to settle down to sleep, and then I noticed that I had several missed calls from Rachele, so I called her back. She suggested that I let the hospital know that my waters had broken. This I did not want to do, but I figured I should go along with that.

By now, it's about 3:30 am. So, I called my dad and let him know that it was time for them to come over. He said that they would leave straight away. I also called Rachele and told her the same thing. I came out to the living room, where Arthur was to let him know that I was in labour now and had called everyone. The contractions were coming quick, and I tried to bounce on the ball, which I loved for my first labour, but the ball was too intense during contractions for this labour. I needed to kneel and take a deep breath as soon as I felt a contraction coming on.

I stopped using the app to time contractions, but it was plain to both of us that I was in active labour already. The contractions were close together, intense and lasting long enough to make me really need to concentrate during each breath. As we got all our bags ready and settled down to wait, we discussed back and forth whether we should just leave, knowing that my parents were on their way. I was messaging them back and forth, and when they were 10 minutes away at about 4:40 am, we started to get ready to get out the door and ended up passing them just as they pulled up. I gave them both a quick hug as we got in the car just before 5 am. Arthur was more than a little annoyed that I didn't call them straight away and told me as such as I tried to hold myself together through the car ride. Fortunately, the contractions were still frequent but less intense, even in that uncomfortable position. The labour was definitely more intense than I remember from my first, and while I was only comfortable kneeling on all fours or standing, I manage to survive the 40-minute car trip alright.

At the hospital, I tried to get myself organised, have the bath filled, and get my things together, but it was so hard with the contractions coming and coming. Rachele arrived, looking somewhat put out also, and got herself sorted. I find out later that she had her own encounter with the awful desk lady.

The hospital midwife eventually came in and explained that she had to be there and had a long speech about her legal requirements (and I'm just like, "Don't care. Contractions"). I'm guessing she felt weird being there with Rachele and wasn't sure what her role was. She asked me to let her know when there's a space in my contractions so she can palp my tummy and strap the wireless monitor on. I tell her that they're back-to-back, and Rachele asks why she can't do it with me on the floor there, and she replies that she needs to feel for the baby's position too.

Eventually, I had a short window where I could get on the bed. I had been planning to refuse the monitor but decided at that moment to just agree and make them happy. It was so much easier than arguing and I didn't even notice it was there. She went to whisper something to Rachele, and I yell at her to hurry up because I have hardly any pain-free window, and I'm scared about having a contraction lying down. I got back down on all fours as soon as she finished, and by then, I was making groaning noises with each contraction, clinging on to the fit ball and telling anyone who would listen that the ball wasn't working.

The hospital midwife, by then, started a new speech about how I should have the strep B swab (which I had not had obviously on purpose). What on earth she thought I would need that for at this stage of active labour was anyone's guess. I then needed to tune her voice out completely, as she hadn't said anything useful yet and I had no mental energy to engage with her. A few minutes later, she started to say that they recommended a cannula and I say, loudly and clearly, "no cannula!" I didn't hear another peep from her.

I didn't know it at the time, but I went through transition at this time as I laboured on the floor. I felt it as a flash of fear. I wanted to tell everyone that I was afraid, but I decided not to, as I didn't want to hear their responses. It was short lived, and I asked if I could get in the bath, and they said yes. I stood up to get my rash shirt on that Arthur handed me while I leaned on the bed. I started to feel myself needing to push and I knew that this was my last chance to get in that bath. It was such a strange feeling, like needing to throw up but coming out of my vagina. My legs buckled with the force of the involuntary push, and I made a weird noise, like some kind of wild animal call. It was clear that I was in the second stage. I started to calculate. It seemed unlikely that I could make it to the bath. By the time I got my pants off, they would surely be able to see something coming out. I could definitely feel it in my vagina. I keep making the strange wailing sound involuntarily with each contraction, but they were no longer painful at all.

I made a decision and I said that the baby is coming. I wasn't fooling anyone by getting in the pool now, pretending I wasn't pushing. Rachele helped me get my tracky dacks and grandma nappy off while the reception nurse and others start arguing about which doctor on duty to call, Jane or Chris. Someone asks me where I feel the pressure, in my bum or vagina, and I say, "vagina." I definitely never felt that need to poo that everyone talks about. I started pushing with the next couple of contractions and feel something start to come out. I brace myself for the pressure you're supposed to feel in your bum and stretching of the perineum, but I didn't feel that at all but what I'm pushing gets lower and lower, until what I am pushing flicks out and I can hear Rachele talking about the presenting part, which I can feel is one long leg hanging out of me. Through my fog, I realise numbly that I had pushed out a knee and now a whole leg. My midwife took photos of this, and from that I saw that this was his whole left leg right up to the upper thigh.

Dr. Jane, the registrar on duty, came in at some point, and told me it was time to get on the bed with my legs in stirrups, which is exactly what I was told would NOT happen and I would not be asked to do, so I ignored the instruction and kept standing there, listening to my body calmly and waiting to feel more pushing contractions. Fortunately, Rachele was there. She told me it was alright; the leg has been out too long, and they needed to get the other one out. I listened to her and got up on the bed, crawling on all fours with this leg hanging out of me. Such a strange feeling! But I was calm, and steadily got my legs up in the stirrups and laid back.

At this point, quite without warning, let alone consent, Jane reached her hand inside me, and I yelled, “Ow, ow, ow! Stop,” which she did, and I see her face then, for the first time. She looked rattled, like she was trying to be as calm as possible and explains to me that she has to get the other leg out. Rachele echoes this and calmly explains that they need the baby out quickly now. She later explained that, while the baby was not in any obvious danger, his heart rate was starting to dip with the contractions, and they were wanting him out sooner rather than later, given he wasn’t bum first as expected. I agreed, and Jane reached in again. I yelled out again but didn’t tell her to stop and felt the other leg flicking down. This hurt a lot, and I believe that this was the source of my second-degree tear, as I didn’t feel any pain, or even any sensation, after this.

Once both legs were out, Chris, who I noticed was also there between my legs, started telling me to push, and this was echoed by some of the other people around my bed who I was only vaguely aware of. I ignored this, as I knew to only push during contractions and only when I felt like pushing, which I did not feel again after that first leg was out. I had a few more contractions, which I only knew was happening because I made that strange wailing sound, but I had no idea what I was feeling, and I didn’t push consciously.

Dr. Jane later came to visit and explained more about what happened down her end; that the baby was lying sideways in the birth canal, and she had righted his body when she reached inside to pull out the other leg. With each contraction, she then performed what is known as the breech manoeuvre, which she had learned from Dr. Smith. This involved pulling the baby out by gently pulling them out, manoeuvring them one way and then another during the contraction while the mother pushed. Once I was up on the bed, she had the end lowered so that she could get up close and make use of gravity, which is so important during breech births. I was glad to hear this, because I had not been aware of this at the time and had wondered how she could let the baby hang if I was up on the bed like that.

Lying there with my legs in the stirrups, I was reminded of my Nana's stories of giving birth like that in the 60s, and even then, could kind of see the funny side of being in exactly that some position 60 years later, after feeling so superior about how I was going to birth my babies. Rachele was on my left side, and I was listening for her voice and encouragement while Arthur was on my right. He looked down briefly and told me that it was a boy (it had been a surprise gender) and he looked so happy and excited that I smiled back, even though it was all so intense at that point. It also reminded me of my dad's birth and how the doctor had told my Nana his gender as she started pushing.

Dr. Jane then told Chris to get the local anaesthetic ready for the episiotomy to get the head out. I had no idea that at this point the body was hanging out of me, because I honestly hadn't felt a thing and had not been consciously pushing. I said, "What?" as Chris went to get the giant scissors that looked to me like garden shears. She held them between my legs and asked if she had my permission. "No!" I screamed.

Rachele reassured me that it was alright, because the baby needed to be born quickly. I asked Alex if it was going to hurt, and she assured me that I would only feel a pulling sensation. I agreed, but watching Chris cut under Jane's direction was scary. Fortunately, I didn't feel anything. I was so shocked later to learn that my baby was hanging out of me by his head at that point. With the next contraction, I made the wailing noise and Chris told me to concentrate on pushing, not yelling, so I closed my mouth and pushed where I assumed the pressure should be and in the next moment my giant 4.2 kg baby was splattered on my chest, angry crying, covered in meconium all over his body, and his head was bright red with my blood. I was so shocked, as even though I knew that he must be nearly out, because I couldn't feel any sensations, I just wasn't ready to have a baby on me. Everyone gasped because he was so big, but he just looked normal to me.

My first thought was, "ewww! Gross!" because of all the blood and poo, and I wanted him wiped down or something. In the next moment, Chris had clamped and then cut the cord cut (without my permission). She took him to the warmer to check him briefly in the room before wiping him down, wrapping him up, and putting him back on my chest. It all happened so quick, and I was so shocked that I didn't think much of it until later, when Arthur remarked that I had not had the chance to cut the cord, which had been my preference. I assume that the unusual position, the meconium, and the less-than-ideal heart rate had been the justification for this, as the whole pushing phase had only lasted 18 minutes, and he certainly appeared to be totally healthy.

As I held my new son, I heard Rachele let them know that I wanted a physiological third stage. They turned to me and asked if that was true. Like most new mums, I had completely forgotten about the placenta while I held my baby. I said, "yes," I wanted a physiological third stage, and then without warning, Chris felt my belly for a second before elbowing me hard like a pro wrestler. I yelled, "ow!" and then Alex pulled on the cord and instructed me to push, which I did, and out squelched the placenta in the next moment.

Looking back, I found this so funny, as even though I can concede that this, and Alex reaching inside me without permission, was obstetric violence, it all resulted in such a good outcome, and I was already feeling such a natural high that I could only laugh about it.

The whole birth from my waters breaking to that moment was just less than 5 hours, with actual labour less than 4 hours. Jasper was born about 50 minutes after we arrived. The worst part was definitely having stitches, as it's still quite painful, even with the local anaesthetic. The gas just makes you more amenable and helps you see the funny side. I was told I wasn't breathing in the gas properly, but I maintain that that's because I couldn't breathe deeply and squeal at the same time.

Once everything was finished, I latched Jasper to the breast easily and I have been exclusively breastfeeding since then and cannot describe what a miracle that is to me after having to exclusively express and formula-feed with my first.

Jasper weighed in at 4.2 kg, 59 cm long, and 37.5 cm head circumference. He was much larger than the scans predicted and yet, he came out so fast, it made me wonder what all the fuss is about with breech birth. Yes, he needed some manoeuvring, but the whole labour was so short and painless, with the exception of when his leg was pulled out and the stitches afterwards.

While I could have gone home immediately, I decided to accept the offer to stay for 24-hour observation due to meconium (which was laughable, considering that Jasper pooed outside the birth canal before his head was born). It meant my husband could get some rest at home and let my parents go home for rest too, and he could get ready for us there. The hospital stay was also nice in its own way, as I got to see how good even a hospital stay can be when you're not stuck lying on your back, unable to move after major surgery while somehow expected also to be learning to look after a newborn. All the midwives made a big deal about how amazing I was to have had a breech VBAC and to be breastfeeding. The whole hospital experience was incredibly redeeming, and I have found myself looking back on my first birth with more acceptance rather than pain and anger.

Again, I can't emphasise enough how wonderful I felt after this birth. Even with the painful stitches. I would find myself laughing at myself affectionately if I couldn't sit for too long. When my milk came in, I cried happy tears, as I thought about how grateful I felt at how everyone had looked after me and allowed me to have this birth. I had no idea it was possible to feel so good physically and mentally after having a baby. I have transformed as a person and started a new and exciting phase of my life.

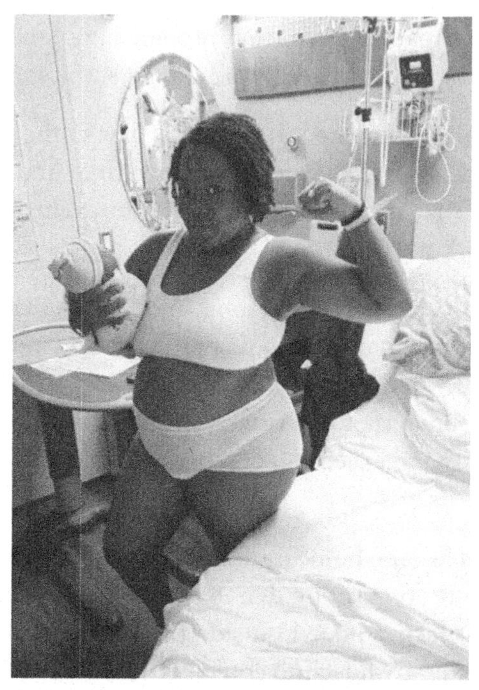

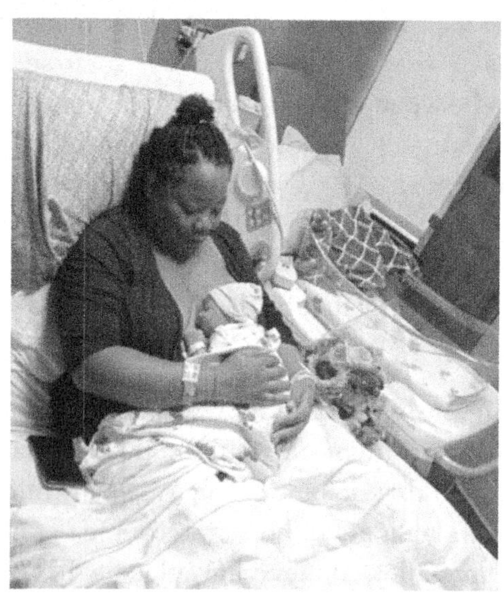

Jasmine, USA

Jasmine – VBAC

After being disappointed that my doctor wanted me to be induced 3 weeks early, the universe aligned itself something wonderful, y'all! With less than a 20% chance of having a successful VBAC because of my age, weight, and race, I got to 10cm after 21 hours, and I pushed my 2nd baby boy out. It only took me about 4 solid pushes and in 8 minutes flat, he was on my chest. I delivered at Vidant Medical in Greenville, North Carolina. My induction was with Pitocin and a foley bulb. My entire team of doctors and nurses were of African American descent and amazing! I feel so special, strong, and powerful! Let me tell you something; being a mother is like no other. My husband, Delroy, almost passed out as soon as he saw the head crowning, and he told me I better hire a photographer if we ever have anymore, because he could barely get any good pics or video of the birth, since he felt dizzy and couldn't believe his eyes, but hey, here's some pics in my sexy postpartum diaper glory, and my labor and delivery socks that were in my @ohbabyboxes package.

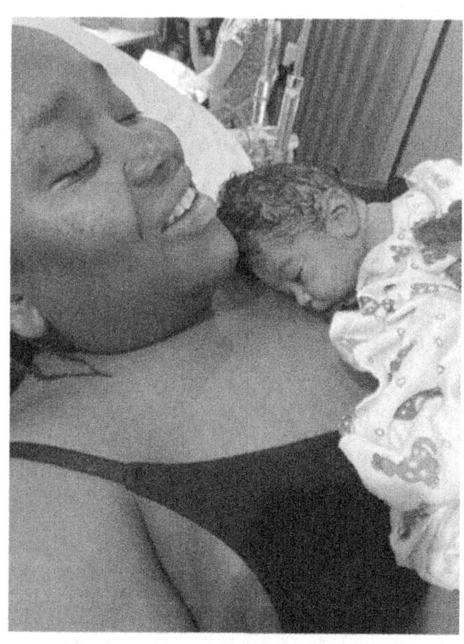

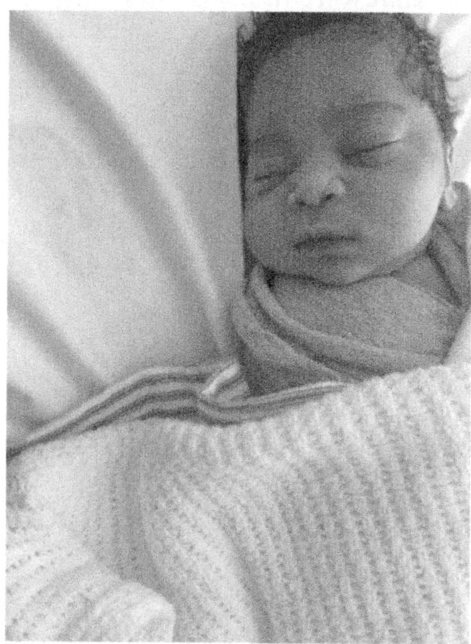

Jemila, Western Australia, Australia

Jemila – VBAC

I had a successful vaginal birth after caesarean section (VBAC) at King Edward Memorial Hospital (KEMH) and I am happy with the outcome, albeit needing an episiotomy and vacuum-assisted delivery.

My first birth was at Albany Regional hospital in January 2019. I had flank pain that was unrelated to my pregnancy, and as I went to my local hospital in Katanning, WA, they quickly sent me to Albany via ambulance. Katanning is a regional hospital with a fully equipped maternity section, which they could not operate due to reasons I am unaware of. All women of that area are to be sent to either Perth, Narrogin, or Albany.

I was only 38 weeks at the time and my baby was nowhere near ready to come, but despite evidence discouraging unnecessary CTG monitoring and interventions, when I went in, a cascade of interventions was made – baby monitoring, induction of labour, epidural; you name it. I was not informed and had not done any adequate research. I had not had good prenatal care due to being remote and simply not being aware of available services in Australia. I have no family in Australia and therefore, was not aware of all the services available, such as the midwifery care program. I saw a midwife for the first time when I was 36 weeks. I did a bit of reading but had somewhat expected that I would be provided or referred to services. I did attend a prenatal class, where the midwife warned that the earlier we go to the hospital, the more "prodding" will occur, which will likely lead to a caesarean section.

So, when I got to the hospital, I thought that they would investigate the flank pain, resolve it, and allow me to go in spontaneous labour but instead, the CTG monitoring identified some distress in the baby's heart rate.

The care itself was wonderful and it's a wonderful hospital with great staff, but my obstetrician (OB) had to bring in a consultant. This consultant, I later found out, was allegedly specialised in gynaecology. He came in at my weakest to offer an epidural, and told me that the latest evidence has shown that induction is not likely to increase my risk of having a caesarean section but decrease my risk of having a caesarean section. He played on my ignorance, and instead of giving me information, I felt that he used his position of power to scare me towards all the interventions.

I was induced due to low variability of the foetal heart (not sure what that means or that I got it right), I progressed to 9cm dilated, but the baby's head was high, and both bub and I were tachycardic. I was spiking high temperatures and therefore, we had to go for a caesarean section. I remember refusing to consent to the c-section and the obstetrician telling me that even though we were an equipped hospital, they were not equipped enough and had to do the section in case we needed a paediatrician, or we would have to be sent to Perth via Royal flying doctor—possibly separately—and that my husband would have to drive to Perth. Things are a bit blurry, but I did end up signing.

My princess was born at 11:26 pm, 38 weeks and 4 days, at 3.56 kg. After she was born, I asked myself what the worry was as she was stable, had normal APGAR, and no need for oxygen or resuscitation. My heart rate went back to normal, and they suspected that the baby was sitting on something leading to my heart working harder to circulate blood. I wondered if a change of position could have fixed this, but I had an epidural so I probably couldn't move. My obstetrician later told me that next time, she would recommend me for a VBAC, since I progressed so well.

I held on to that piece of information and asked her at my 6-week visit about it. She explained that I would need to wait at least 18 months before falling pregnant again. I knew then I would go for a VBAC, but I swore not to return there.

This time around, I started researching as soon as I fell pregnant. I had waited 2 years to fall pregnant and would have this baby 2 years and 10 months after my c-section. It was more than sufficient time to improve my chance for a VBAC. I had moved town but still could not birth locally, as the local hospital did not offer VBAC. I honestly find it sad that women must travel miles from their place of residence just to give birth. I had the option to go back to Albany, Armadale, or KEMH. I would be part of a shared care where I would see my local OB every 6 weeks, my local midwife, and the KEMH OB in late pregnancy.

I not only researched VBAC but I also did a Lamaze VBAC course and watched YouTube videos for exercises to induce labour but joining the WA VBAC Facebook group was probably the best thing I did. I also had acupuncture at 39.1 for my sciatica.

My first appointment at KEMH was positive. The obstetrician asked me what my plans were and provided me with some information. She concluded that I had a low-risk pregnancy and booked the next appointment at 39 weeks. I had to see my local OB in between for monitoring. When I saw my local OB at 38 weeks, she was concerned about my fundal height and suggested I go for an ultrasound. I was worried that they would suggest a c-section due to a large baby or other reasons, so I declined the ultrasound. At 39 weeks, we had the appointment, and KEMH OB offered a Vaginal Examination (VE) and Stretch and Sweep (SS). I learnt from the VBAC group that this was not necessary and had read a paper on it, so I declined. I had been stressing about declining because, culturally, we don't say no to people of authority, especially doctors. I was relieved when my OB was so understanding and said that we could reassess at the next appointment, and we scheduled another appointment at 40 weeks, 2 days.

I went into spontaneous labour at 39 weeks, 5 days at 3 am. I laboured at home for as long as I could. When I rang the hospital, they also encouraged me to stay home but to come in if I felt I needed to. I couldn't by 9:30 am, as they were 2 minutes apart, and went in, got there at 10 am, and explained that I wanted minimal intervention, intermittent monitoring, and limited VE. We did one VE there. A midwife could feel my membranes but confirmed that I was in active labour, and we waited for a birth suite to be ready.

When I got to the labour suite, I continued to refuse constant monitoring and VE, but my labour stalled. I agreed to another VE, and we found my membranes in the way and the midwife could not properly ascertain how dilated I was. She had to bring in OB and a consultant who came in with three options, 1. Do nothing, 2. Break membranes and check dilation plus add oxytocin drip, and 3. Repeat caesarean section. I think there was talk of getting an epidural and canula amongst those options. When trying to explain why my labour would have stalled, the consultant asked me where I am from, as the midwife had suggested something about me being of African descent and the shape of our uterus. I had just read a paper about implicit bias and racism in research the previous day and refuted that. I declined the epidural and sucked on gas as if my life depended on it. I agreed to break my membranes but declined the drip as it was explained to me that it would increase the risk of uterine rupture.

As soon as the OB did the VE, I lost my membranes and we found there was meconium inside. That outcome freaked me out and I stopped fighting a bit. I agreed to the foetal monitoring, and we noticed some deceleration in bubs heart rate but changed position and found one position that he liked. It was 5 pm, I was only 4 cm dilated at that point, and we decided to do another VE in 2 to 3 hours, then reassess. I quickly dilated to 10 cm and was ready to push by 8 pm (I wished I had let them break my membranes when I came in).

As I pushed, bub was having decelerations again and his head was not coming out. We found out that he was posterior and needed some assistance to come out, as they were concerned about the decelerations and meconium. I was so tired by that point and agreed to the episiotomy and vacuum-assisted delivery. I was also concerned about the health of my baby.

My handsome boy was born at 8:37 pm, and let out a small cry. We could not do delayed cord clamping because of the meconium. He had to be seen by the paediatric team (which wasn't a must for me), but they put him straight on me before he was whisked away for peds to do a meconium check. He was safely in my arms again a few minutes later. We are both did but had to stay in hospital for a few days to monitor the baby's head due to a hematoma from the vacuum. Given there was no specialist in my town (two-and-a-half-hour drive away), they erred on the side of caution to prevent us from having to turn around.

If I was to have another child next time, I would ensure that I engage a doula, private midwife, or private OB. It was so exhausting to have to go through labour and be my advocate. My husband supported me, but he had done little to no research. Even though I had done the research, there are things that I was not so sure about and that made me slightly unsure of my decisions.

Having another professional who is health literate would have been a better experience for me. I have always thought that it didn't matter, and I would not get the extra insurance, but now I see how it would have been important. I also did not click with my midwife, and I believe that this personality clash, or whatever it is, created a bit of stress for me. But then, I wonder what it is like for people less privileged (being able to read, able to afford private health cover), who are potentially being unnecessarily being put through labour intervention that could have otherwise been avoided.

I am, however, grateful for the team that looked after me. I challenged them I think with my stubbornness, but they informed me and allowed me to make my decisions. I am also grateful to live in such a great country with an excellent health system (yes, I know there are a few flaws), where I have a say and can question a professional's opinion and obtain an answer instead of being shouted at. I know I wouldn't be able to pull that stint in my country of birth.

I said during labour, "It takes a special person to deal with people in labour and then their babies afterwards." I was referring to the midwives. Gosh, they got their hands full with us. Cheers to the midwives, obstetricians, paediatrician, and every professional working to keep us safe during and after birth. Cheers to us all parents; it takes incredible strength (mental and physical) to labour and birth. Cheers to the Western Australian VBAC group; without the great support, I'm not sure how I would have done.

Laura – Healing VBAC with Lotus Birth

At first, I want to express my limitless gratitude to my beautiful, healthy body, my womb, and my divine daughters while writing this important story about my natural birth in 2020 after having a belly birth in 2018.

In 2018, after 20 hours of labour and being peaceful at home in my love bubble with my husband while being one with the sensations of the waves of the contractions, we ended up in the hospital. I manifested a natural home birth and it looked like it was about to happen. My water broke naturally, and my dilation was progressing naturally until I was about 8 cm. I was so calm and in tune with myself, and ready to meet our creation of love. My husband was ready to catch his baby with bare hands. Then, our midwife told us our baby might be sunny side up. A sunny-side-up baby is a baby positioned head down but facing Mom's abdomen, so the baby's occipital bone (the skull) is against the back of your pelvis. If I must believe the internet, only 5 to 8% of babies are in sunny side-up position. Still, I was calm and empowered because I did a lot of research prior to childbirth. The midwife said, "When you feel the urge to push, I will guide you through it because your baby isn't in the most ideal position." Since I was so exhausted after being in labour for 20 hours, the midwife suggested I go to the hospital.

It felt like the earth stood still because this wasn't planned. But I shifted my energy directly and looked at my husband, and we just went with the flow. Being in the hospital (still no epidural or medicine), I pushed for 3 hours straight, and each time it felt like my baby came out a bit and then went back. I gave everything I had. I was exhausted, and then, the doctors had to quickly shift, and told us that because of the long hours and safety for the baby and me, an emergency c-section (or how I like to call it, "belly birth") was necessary. I honestly had no time to process this information, since we were already in the elevator to go to the operation room. As a matter of fact, I was still pushing in the elevator, and even when the anaesthetist tried to give me the epidural, I couldn't stop the force of nature.

Bright lights were shining in my eyes while I was laying in the operation room. I looked in the eyes of my husband and I had to trust the doctors completely. Then, in what felt like an hour, but I think it was only 20 minutes, there she was, eventually, my beautiful baby goddess. I was so incredibly happy! She is here!

Being a new mother, you are in autopilot mode; everything is new and beautiful but also hard, and you are undergoing a whole new transformation as a woman. So, after a couple of months, when my daughter was already a little bit older, I found the time to feel what I was feeling, and I had to heal myself and accept my body with the belly birth scar and the soft belly. I was so close with birthing my daughter the natural way, that I felt I failed myself and my daughter. I mean, like, her head was almost out! It felt so frustrating to think about it! Later on, while healing my birth trauma, I learned more about sunny side up babies and I know that I did everything I could. even the doctors said that. So, I felt at peace and grateful for my experience.

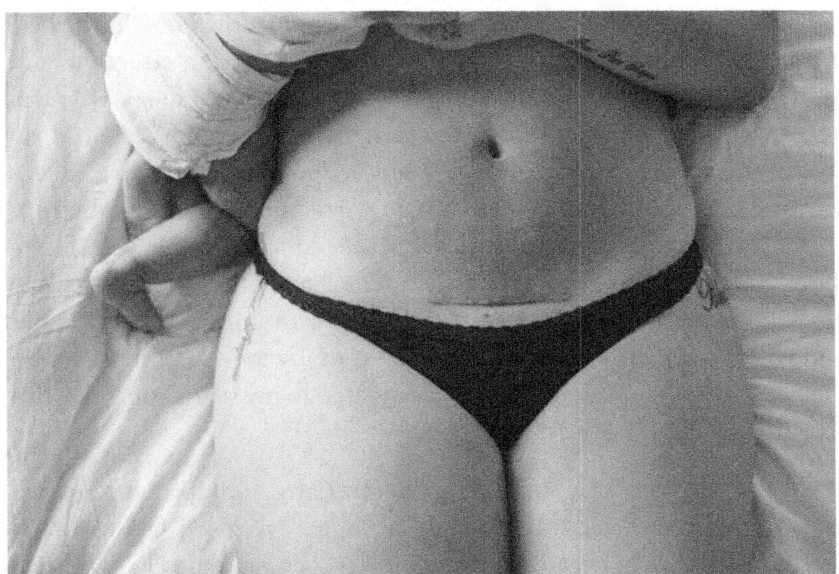

After 2.5 years, when I welcomed another star seed in my womb, I was determined to give birth naturally. I talked and trusted the midwife and I shared my story, my fears of the rupturing scar, and complications but also my manifestation of giving birth naturally. She was so supportive, and I totally felt confident to do it. I talked to my baby in my womb, I

read Ina Maya's *Guide to Childbirth* again, as well as another hypnobirthing book, and I was totally prepared for giving divine birth.

Then, at 36 weeks, the midwife felt that my baby was breech. When I heard that my divine baby was in breech position, it gave me anxiety because it is not the most ideal position for our baby to be born, especially when your first birth experience was a belly birth. It was really confronting, and pointed me directly back to my healing, and shadow work. I was holding myself together and accepted and observed all the emotions that I was feeling. I felt more comfortable by not sharing this news with my family, and I only wanted to deal with it with my husband, Ray, because I was determined to turn our divine star seed myself. On Tuesday, we received the news, and after I got my emotional, hormonal self together, I started doing different exercises, combined with meditating to make more room in my divine womb, and to open my lower pelvis.

If you look up on YouTube how doctors try to turn the baby in the best birth position, it is uncomfortable. Plus, if you have a c-section scar, there will be a lot of pressure on your scar, so it's not ideal. One day, before we were supposed to go to the hospital, Ray and I tried Moxa therapy (traditional Chinese medicine acupuncture), which consists burning herbs and applying the heat on particular points of the body to let the Yang energy flow (in this case, directed to my lower pelvis). We didn't have a special Moxa stick, so Ray came up with the idea to use my black tourmaline massage stick and heat it with hot water. I was calm, and with Ray holding the hot crystal next to my toes, I connected with the baby, asked him/her to turn, and directed to my sacred portal. I also repeatedly said, "Relax, release, open."

The morning after, I could feel that my baby had turned. and the midwife also confirmed it. What an absolute overjoyed feeling of joy and an abundance of gratitude! I felt even more than ready to give birth naturally/vaginally.

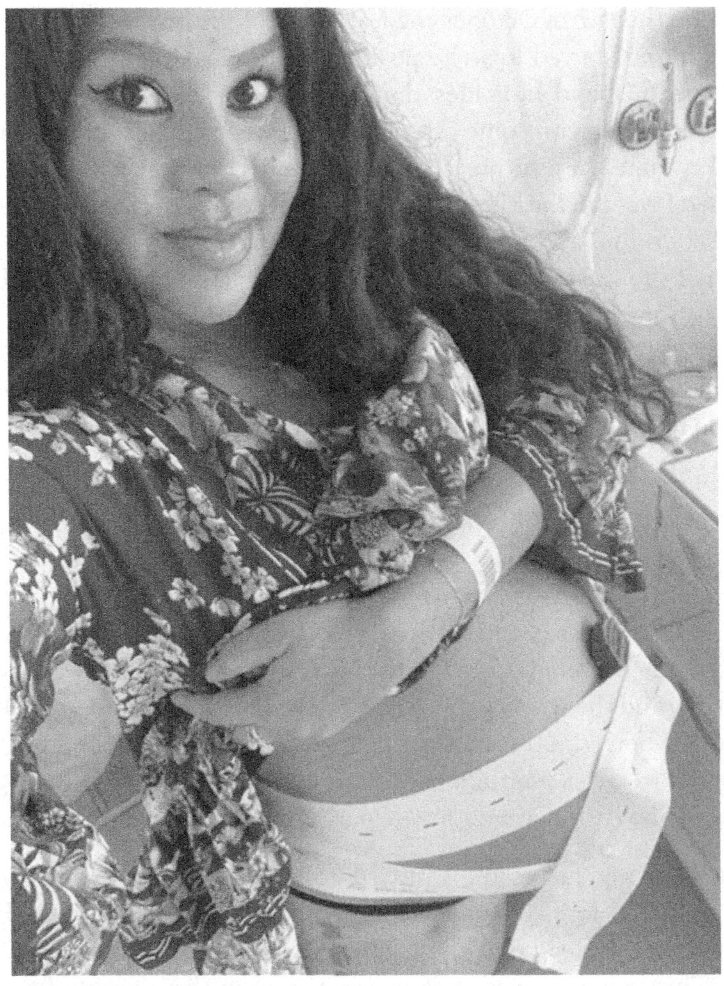

Then, at 41 weeks and 5 days, I started having light contractions. I wanted to birth at home, but because of my belly birth history, the midwifes suggested that I had to give birth in the hospital so that they could safely monitor the pressure on my scar. I agreed, but it was an absolute must for me to move during contractions. So, the hospital especially arranged a mobile monitor belly belt for me so that I could move and go in out of the birthing pool, and that I could have the birth of my dreams.

Then, on the 12th of October 2020, at around 5 pm, my water broke. I was so calm and started to write positive birth affirmations in my journal while my husband and oldest daughter set up the birthing pool and put on the diffuser with some essential oils so that the hospital room felt a bit like home. At 6:30 pm, the waves of my contractions started to get heavier. I went in the birthing pool, but it felt too cramped. So, I decided to walk around and to go into the shower so that the only water could channel the waves of the contractions. So, at around 10 pm, when my contractions were at the heaviest, the doctor kindly asked if I could lay down so she could see how far I was. I was calm and in tune with the contractions, and ready to meet my baby. I pushed a couple of times, and I could feel my baby lower in my pelvis. It was really happening!

At around 10:40 pm, it was burning. Was this the ring of fire? I was so clear in my mind and full of adrenaline, and I could hear the midwife saying, "Hold it, your baby is about to be born." Then, I had to wait to for another correction to push my baby out. My yoni was burning like never before! Then, at 10:45 pm, one final push, where my husband catches our 2nd daughter with his bare hands. I was so happy and in awe of myself, my baby, and the whole experience. I was completely euphoric. I did it! I did it! My body did this in less than 3.5 hours! At that point, I promised to myself to never ever talk bad about my body again or to be negative about my belly or scar and so on. I am a beautiful, powerful mother!

Because of my successful VBAC, I could also have the lotus birth I dreamed of. A lotus birth is when the umbilical cord is left attached to the placenta, instead of being clamped and cut until it falls away on its own. This means the baby stays connected to the placenta for longer than with a typical birth. Like delayed cord clamping, a lotus birth doesn't disrupt blood volume and allows the oxygenated blood to flow back into the baby. This improves blood circulation, body temperature, red blood cell count, the immune system, and brain development. It resonates with me, so it was also beautiful for me to experience it.

This was not only the birth of another healthy, beautiful, big, baby girl but also a rebirth for me as a mother, a woman, and a womb goddess!

To all birthing mommas, you are amazingly beautiful! Powerful! And I see you! Trust your body and baby. Sending limitless love to all mommas!

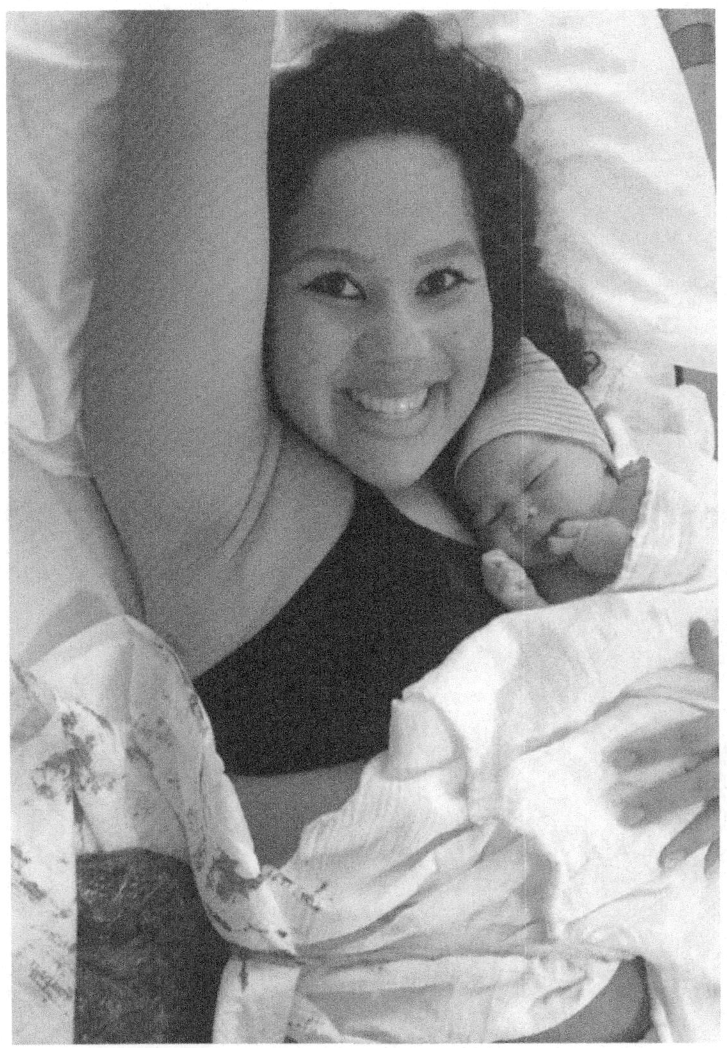

Laura-Zofia Rosales, Amsterdam, The Netherlands

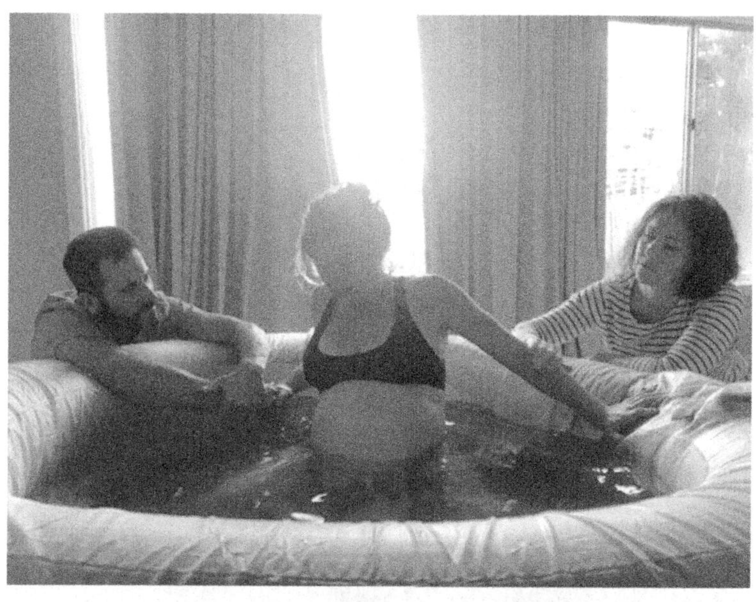

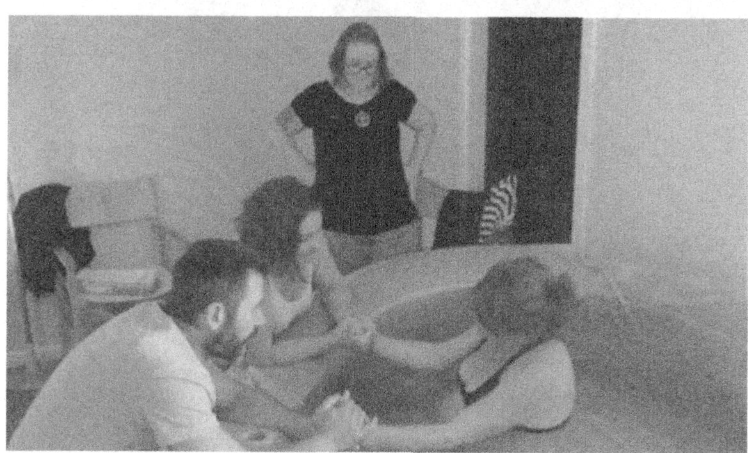

Sasha Cody, NSW, Australia

Podcast episode: https://themotherhoodcircle.com.au/sasha-hba2c/

Sasha – Homebirth after 2 Caesareans

My first birth was the opposite of what I expected. To say I had a rosy view of birth is an understatement. Growing up as a horse breaker/ trainer, and in later years, being a performing aerial acrobat, I have a high comfort level with my body's strength. Also, a deep trust in its physical capabilities, a trust that is essential to both horse breaking and acrobatics. Added to all of this, I grew up hearing how my mum laboured 3 hours with both my sister and I and was back on her feet that afternoon in both cases.

I confidently went through all the normal processes of signing up with a GP and going to our local public hospital for the birth of Billy. The first obstacle was pushing past all the necessary induction moments. This happened on the due date, then at 41 weeks, and then at 10 days, until they reluctantly agreed to let me try for 40+12. I was spoken to in ways I would never have tolerated by my 3rd birth, by which point, I knew who was really the boss (me).

That labour was long. I wasn't prepared for the pain and pressure, and tired myself out too early with all of my active birth techniques. I saw every midwife in the hospital as the shifts changed and the doctors were busy in and out. Never had any baby stress but it was just a long time. As I grew more exhausted (and agreed to the epidural and then continued to labour), the language in the room changed. The doctors took a more front and centre role, and I faded into the background, becoming more apologetic about the inconvenience I felt I was. It wasn't hard for them to undermine me and turn me on my back and take away my last shreds of strength and hopes for a natural birth.

That was one heartbreak that was always going to be there for me, but the other came from the subsequent treatment. The dismissive talk from the doctor, the clumsy crashing of the hospital bed in the corridor with me desperately catching my own catheter bag, the lack of care, and the annoyance at my fear while I lay there paralysed with spinal block; these things all added another layer to my well-rounded devastation and disappointment at Billy's birth.

Falling pregnant again with Bobby, my first thought was joy, which then galloped quickly towards despair at how the hell was this birth going to happen. Did I have to have a c-section? Did I have a chance to try again? I was led to believe no from my conversations with the midwives and doctors. I would have to have another c-section.

Then, I found Hazel. I rang her, she listened, and I poured it out. She turned my confidence back around in that one phone call. I was the one in charge. I could do what I wanted. We planned a home birth. I obsessed over it. It was to be the opposite of hospital. Outside in a birth pool, amongst the trees on our property. The set up was beautiful, the lead up gentle and unhurried, and again, the labour started late but naturally. Again, we laboured long, and being an hour away from hospital, we made the tough but safer decision to transfer. A real part of any home birth plan.

With my wonderful and famous midwife by my side, we entered the hospital in a different way. We were treated with so much grace and respect that, although the birth was by c-section again, we had a different feeling and experience. We had done what we could, and I had made the decisions.

Surprise pregnancy number 3! Surely now, I was out of birth options. Not so. Hazel, again, told me I could do what I wanted. So a home birth was planned again. This time, we rented a house near the hospital, and I also lied a bit about my period so that I could buy myself some extra days to let the baby come in its own time: a healthy pregnancy, like the first ones. Minimal appointments suited me just fine. Life was normal. I was much less obsessive about statistics and reading the entire internet, like I had been with the previous planned homebirth. My only plan this time was telling my support crew, "Don't let me give up."

The labour was the same, long and slow. I was ready for it this time, though. Lots of rest, snacks, and simple breathing techniques. I wanted to give up many times. I begged for an epidural. I second guessed myself and asked for a bazillion examinations, but Hazel knew me. Not only had she seen me the entire pregnancy, but for the previous one too. She knew me as strong and fit. She knew my feelings to the core. She knew my medical history. Mostly, she knew to listen and trust. "I want to give up," I would say. "You're okay, baby's okay. Let's give it a bit longer," she said, crafty and wise, cool and calm, managing her demeanour, even when there were some moments of concern, which is more than I can say for the hospital staff. I felt safer and that my unborn baby was safer with Hazel than I did in the hospital setting. I think this was because I was more switched on instinctively (as opposed to switched off) in this company and environment compared to hospital.

I doubted the baby would come out until his head was in my hand. It was a 20-hour labour (again) and we did it on our own. We would never have been given that time in hospital, and certainly would not have been given the option of the birth pool, which was the only reason I coped with the pain, and there wouldn't have been all those stairs to climb up and down to get things moving either.

Even if Hazel had have come with me to hospital, she would have been sidelined and unable to be the primary person for me to lean on and listen to throughout. I could hear her in the distance during labour, at the back of my contractions, and when I'd open my eyes for a glimpse of the outside world around me. I understood her and knew what she meant from a few words, and she understood my mutterings. I didn't have to be introduced to a million different people and specialists walking in and out of the room. We were in tune, as mother and midwife.

I understand the hospital setting, and I am grateful for its lifesaving capabilities. I know that things can go badly with birth quickly too. I obviously heard it all, being a VBAC2C pregnant lady. I read and understood all the risks. But I would, in a heartbeat, do it this way again. I think it is the safest option in the setting that we have available to us in Australia. I'm so glad I didn't have to try and recover after a 3rd c-section. I'm so glad I met Hazel.

I'm devastated for all the women who won't meet a Hazel and who have to then convince themselves and sign up to the subscribed belief that surgical birth and heavily medicalised birth is what's best for the baby or accept something because "the doctor won't let me," and "as long as you have a healthy baby, that's all that matters." I'm at the age where

I have watched several of my friends hang up their baby-having hat with those parting thoughts and feelings around birth. Tragic, but also bullshit.

I'm one of the lucky few in this world to have met Hazel and had her at my births. I wish there were more Hazels in Australia for other women birthing but for that to happen, things need to change in a big way.

FINAL THOUGHTS

This book has been a joy to write. I have really loved diving into the recent research on lots of different topics and sharing my VBAC research with you. I am also so grateful to the women who eagerly shared their stories from across the world in this book. Thank you for reading this book and I wish you well on your better-birth experience.

As a midwife and a researcher, I believe that you can have a better birth and that the four factors of control confidence, relationship, and active labour are pivotal in you achieving that better-birthing experience.

Please come and find me on Facebook and Instagram at Hazel Keedle VBAC researcher. https://www.facebook.com/VBACmatters

I love hearing from women who have had a better birth after a previous caesarean so please do drop me a message and let me know how you achieved your better birth!

References

ACOG. (2017). *Practice Bulletin No. 184 Vaginal Birth After Cesarean Delivery*. I. Wolters Kluwer Health. https://www.acog.org/Womens-Health/Vaginal-Birth-After-Cesarean-VBAC

Adams, C., & Curtin-Bowen, M. (2021). Countervailing powers in the labor room: The doula-doctor relationship in the United States. *Soc Sci Med, 285*, 114296. https://doi.org/10.1016/j.socscimed.2021.114296

AIHW. (2020). *Australia's mothers and babies 2018—in brief.*

Akhavan, S., & Edge, D. (2012). Foreign-born women's experiences of community-based doulas in Sweden—A qualitative study. *Health Care for Women International, 33*(9), 833-848. https://doi.org/10.1080/07399332.2011.646107

Alfirevic, Z., Gyte, G. M. L., Cuthbert, A., & Devane, D. (2017). Continuous cardiotocography (CTG) as a form of electronic fetal monitoring (EFM) for fetal assessment during labour. *Cochrane database of systematic reviews*(2). https://doi.org/10.1002/14651858.CD006066.pub3 (Cochrane Database of Systematic Reviews)

Amiri, B. (2020). Reproductive abuse is rampant in the immigration detention system. *American Civil Liberties Union*. https://www.aclu.org/news/immigrants-rights/reproductive-abuse-is-rampant-in-the-immigration-detention-system/

Anderson, C. A. (2017). The trauma of birth. *Health Care for Women International, 38*(10), 999-1010. https://doi.org/10.1080/07399332.2017.1363208

Andrews, P. (1996). Violence against Aboriginal women in Australia: Possibilities for redress within the international human rights framework. *Albany Law Review, 60*, 917.

APA. (2013). *Diagnostic and statistical manual of mental disorders (DSM-5®)*. American Psychiatric Association.

Asadzadeh, L., Jafari, E., Kharaghani, R., & Taremian, F. (2020). Effectiveness of midwife-led brief counseling intervention on post-traumatic stress disorder, depression, and anxiety symptoms of women experiencing a traumatic childbirth: a randomized controlled trial. *BMC Pregnancy Childbirth, 20*(1). https://doi.org/10.1186/s12884-020-2826-1

Aune, K., & Holyoak, R. (2018). Navigating the third wave: Contemporary UK feminist activists and 'third-wave feminism'. *Feminist Theory, 19*(2), 183-203. https://doi.org/10.1177/1464700117723593

Ayers, S., McKenzie-McHarg, K., & Slade, P. (2015). Post-traumatic stress disorder after birth. *Journal of Reproductive and Infant Psychology, 33*(3), 215-218. https://doi.org/10.1080/02646838.2015.1030250

Ayers, S., Wright, D. B., & Thornton, A. (2018). Development of a measure of postpartum PTSD: The city birth trauma scale. *Frontiers in Psychiatry, 9*. https://doi.org/10.3389/fpsyt.2018.00409

Bakhshi, T., Landon, M. B., Lai, Y., Spong, C. Y., Rouse, D. J., Leveno, K. J., Varner, M. W., Caritis, S. N., Meis, P. J., Wapner, R. J., Sorokin, Y., Miodovnik, M., Carpenter, M., Peaceman, A. M., O'Sullivan, M. J., Sibai, B. M., Langer, O., Thorp, J. M., & Mercer, B. M. (2010). Maternal and neonatal outcomes of repeat cesarean delivery in women with a prior classical versus low transverse uterine incision. *Am J Perinatol, 27*(10), 791-796. https://doi.org/10.1055/s-0030-1254238

Barnett, R. (2005). A horse named 'Twilight Sleep': The language of obstetric anaesthesia in 20th century Britain. *International Journal of Obstetric Anesthesia, 14*(4), 310-315. https://doi.org/10.1016/j.ijoa.2004.12.011

Basavaraddi, I. (2015). *Yoga: Its origin, history and development.* Ministry of External Affairs, Government of India. https://www.mea.gov.in/search-result.htm?25096/Yoga:_su_origen,_historia_y_desarrollo

Bastos, M. H., Furuta, M., Small, R., McKenzie McHarg, K., & Bick, D. (2015). Debriefing interventions for the prevention of psychological trauma in women following childbirth. *Cochrane Database of Systematic Reviews* (4) CD007194. http://doi: 10.1002/14651858.CD007194.pub2.

Baxter, J. (2019). Postnatal debriefing: Women's need to talk after birth. *British Journal of Midwifery, 27*(9), 563-571. https://doi.org/10.12968/bjom.2019.27.9.563

Baxter, J. (2020). An exploration of reasons why some women may leave the birth experience with emotional distress. *British Journal of Midwifery, 28*(1), 24-33. https://doi.org/10.12968/bjom.2020.28.1.24

Baxter, J. D., McCourt, C., & Jarrett, P. M. (2014). What is current practice in offering debriefing services to postpartum women and what are the perceptions of women in accessing these services: A critical review of the literature. *Midwifery, 30*(2), 194-219. https://doi.org/10.1016/j.midw.2013.12.013

Bayrampour, H., Lisonkova, S., Tamana, S., Wines, J., Vedam, S., & Janssen, P. (2021). Perinatal outcomes of planned home birth after cesarean and planned hospital vaginal birth after cesarean at term gestation in British Columbia, Canada: A retrospective population based cohort study. *Birth.* https://doi.org/10.1111/birt.12539

Beck, C. T. (2004). Birth trauma: In the eye of the beholder. *Nursing Research, 53*(1), 28-35.

Beck, C. T. (2017). The anniversary of birth trauma: A metaphor analysis. *Journal of Perinatal Education, 26*(4), 219-228. https://doi.org/10.1891/1058-1243.26.4.219

Beckett, K. (2005). Choosing cesarean: Feminism and the politics of childbirth in the United States. *Feminist Theory, 6*(3), 251-275. https://doi.org/10.1177/1464700105057363

Beckmann, L., Barger, M., Dorin, L., Metzing, S., & Hellmers, C. (2014). Vaginal birth after cesarean in German out-of-hospital settings: Maternal and neonatal outcomes of women with their second child. *Birth.* https://doi.org/10.1111/birt.12130

Behrendt, L. (1993). Aboriginal women and the white lies of the feminist movement: Implications for aboriginal women in rights discourse. *Australian Feminist Law Journal, 1*(1), 27-44. https://doi.org/10.1080/13200968.1993.11077108

Blazkova, B., Pastorkova, A., Solansky, I., Veleminsky, M., Rossnerova, A., Honkova, K., Rossner, P., & Sram, R. J. (2020). The impact of cesarean and vaginal delivery on results of psychological cognitive test in 5 year old children. *Medicina, 56*(10), 554.

Bohren, M. A., Hofmeyr, G. J., Sakala, C., Fukuzawa, R. K., & Cuthbert, A. (2017). Continuous support for women during childbirth. *Cochrane Database of Systematic Reviews, 2017*(8).https://doi.org/10.1002/14651858.cd003766.pub6

Boston Women's Health Collective. (1971). *Our Bodies Our Selves: A Course by and for Women.*

Brown, W. J., Hayman, M., Haakstad, L. A. H., Mielke, G.I., Mena, G.P., Lamerton, T., Green, A., Keating, S.E., Gomes, G.A.O., & Coombes, J.S. (2020). *Evidence-based physical activity guidelines for pregnant women.* Report for the Australian Government Department of Health. https://www.health.gov.au › documents › 2021/0

Buhimschi, C. S., Buhimschi, I. A., Patel, S., Malinow, A. M., & Weiner, C. P. (2005). Rupture of the uterine scar during term labour: contractility or biochemistry? [Comparative Study Multicenter Study Research Support, Non-U.S. Gov't]. *BJOG : An International Journal of Obstetrics and Gynaecology, 112*(1), 38-42. https://doi.org/10.1111/j.1471-0528.2004.00300.x

Bullough, S., Southward, J., & Sharp, A. (2021). Vaginal prostaglandinE2 versus double-balloon catheter for induction of labour for vaginal birth after caesarean section: A retrospective cohort study. *European Journal of Obstetrics, Gynecology, & Reproductive Biology, 259*, 90-94. https://doi.org/10.1016/j.ejogrb.2021.02.007

Byrskog, U., Small, R., & Schytt, E. (2020). Community-based bilingual doulas for migrant women in labour and birth – Findings from a Swedish register-based cohort study. *BMC Pregnancy Childbirth, 20*(1). https://doi.org/10.1186/s12884-020-03412-x

Cahill, A. G., Tuuli, M., Odibo, A. O., Stamilio, D. M., & Macones, G. A. (2010). Vaginal birth after caesarean for women with three or more prior caesareans: Assessing safety and success [Multicenter Study Research Support, N.I.H., Extramural]. *BJOG, 117*(4), 422-427. https://doi.org/10.1111/j.1471-0528.2010.02498.x

Campbell, V., & Nolan, M. (2019). 'It definitely made a difference': A grounded-theory study of yoga for pregnancy and women's self-efficacy for labour. *Midwifery, 68*, 74-83. https://doi.org/10.1016/j.midw.2018.10.005

Carlsson, T., & Ulfsdottir, H. (2020). Waterbirth in low risk pregnancy: An exploration of women's experiences. *Journal of Advanced Nursing, 76*(5), 1221-1231. https://doi.org/10.1111/jan.14336

Chang, Y. H. (2020). Uterine rupture over 11 years: A retrospective descriptive study. *Australian and New Zealand Journal of Obstetrics and Gynaecology, 60*(5), 709-713. https://doi.org/10.1111/ajo.13133

Charter, R., Ussher, J. M., Perz, J., & Robinson, K. (2018). The transgender parent: Experiences and constructions of pregnancy and parenthood for transgender men in Australia. *International Journal of Transgenderism, 19*(1), 64-77. https://doi.org/10.1080/15532739.2017.1399496

Chauhan, S. P., Magann, E. F., Wiggs, C. D., Barrilleaux, P. S., & Martin Jr, J. N. (2002). Pregnancy after classic cesarean delivery. *Obstetrics & Gynecology, 100*(5), 946-950.

Cheyney, M., Bovbjerg, M., Everson, C., Gordon, W., Hannibal, D., & Vedam, S. (2014, Jan-Feb). Outcomes of care for 16,924 planned home births in the United States: the Midwives Alliance of North America Statistics Project, 2004 to 2009. *J Midwifery & Women's Health, 59*(1), 17-27. https://doi.org/10.1111/jmwh.12172

Clark, E. A. S., Silver, R.M. (2011). Long-term maternal morbidity associated with repeat cesarean delivery. *American journal of Obstetrics and Gynecology, 205*(6), S2-S10.

Clews, C., Church, S., & Ekberg, M. (2019). Women and waterbirth: A systematic meta-synthesis of qualitative studies. *Women and Birth, 33*(6), 566-573. https://doi.org/10.1016/j.wombi.2019.11.007

Cohen, N. W., & Estner, L. J. (1983). *Silent knife: Cesarean prevention and vaginal birth after cesarean (VBAC).* Bergin & Garvey.

Cooper, M., & Warland, J. (2019). What are the benefits? Are they concerned? Women's experiences of water immersion for labor and birth. *Midwifery, 79*, 102541. https://doi.org/10.1016/j.midw.2019.102541

Crowther, C., Dodd, J. M., Hiller, J. E., Haslam, R. R., & Robinson, J. S. (2012). Planned vaginal birth or elective repeat caesarean: Patient preference restricted cohort with nested randomised trial. *PLoS Med, 9*(3). https://doi.org/10.1371/journal.pmed.1001192

Dahlen, H. G., Dowling, H., Tracy, M., Schmied, V., & Tracy, S. (2013). Maternal and perinatal outcomes amongst low risk women giving birth in water compared to six birth positions on land. A descriptive cross sectional study in a birth centre over 12 years. *Midwifery, 29*(7), 759-764. https://doi.org/10.1016/j.midw.2012.07.002

Darwin, Z., Green, J., McLeish, J., Willmot, H., & Spiby, H. (2017). Evaluation of trained volunteer doula services for disadvantaged women in five areas in England: Women's experiences. *Health & Social Care in the Community, 25*(2), 466-477. https://doi.org/10.1111/hsc.12331

Davis-Floyd, R. (1993). The technocratic model of birth. *Childbirth: Changing Ideas and Practices in Britain and America 1600 to the Present*, 247-276.

De Campos, E. A., Narchi, N. Z., & Moreno, G. (2020). Meanings and perceptions of women regarding the practice of yoga in pregnancy: A qualitative study. *Complementary Therapies in Clinical Practice, 39*, 101099. https://doi.org/10.1016/j.ctcp.2020.101099

Dejoy, S. B., Bittner, K., & Mandel, D. (2016). A qualitative study of the maternity care experiences of women with obesity: "More than just a number on the scale." *Journal of Midwifery & Women's Health, 61*(2), 217-223. https://doi.org/10.1111/jmwh.12375

Dekker, G. A., Chan, A., Luke, C.G., Priest, K., Riley, M., Halliday, J., King, J.F., Gee, V., O'Neill, M., Snell, M., Cull, V., & Cornes, S. (2010). Risk of uterine rupture in Australian women attempting vaginal birth after one prior caesarean section: A retrospective population-based cohort study. *BJOG: An International Journal of Obstetrics and Gynaecology, 117*, 1358-1365.

Department of Health. (2020). *Clinical practice guidelines: Pregnancy care.* https://www.health.gov.au/resources/pregnancy-care-guidelines

Desisto, C. L., Hirai, A. H., Collins, J. W., & Rankin, K. M. (2018). Deconstructing a disparity: Explaining excess preterm birth among U.S.-born black women. *Annals of Epidemiology, 28*(4), 225-230. https://doi.org/10.1016/j.annepidem.2018.01.012

Dipietro, L., Evenson, K. R., Bloodgood, B., Sprow, K., Troiano, R. P., Piercy, K. L. et al. (2019). Benefits of physical activity during pregnancy and postpartum: An umbrella review. *Medical Science in Sports & Exercise, 51*(6), 1292-1302. https://doi.org/10.1249/MSS.0000000000001941

Dougan, C., Smith, E., Ploski, J., Mc Nally, A., & Johnston, K. (2019). Patients at the centre of care: Debriefing patients after caesarean section. *BMJ Open Quality, 8*(4), e000454. https://doi.org/10.1136/bmjoq-2018-000454

Eley, V. A., Callaway, L., & Van Zundert, A. A. (2015). Developments in labour analgesia and their use in Australia. *Anaesthesia and Intensive Care, 43*(1 suppl), 12-21. https://doi.org/10.1177/0310057x150430s104

England, P., & Horowitz, R. (1998). *Birthing from within: An extra-ordinary guide to childbirth preparation.* Partera Press.

Euro-Peristat Project. (2018). *European Perinatal Health Report: Core indicators of the health and care of pregnant women and babies in Europe in 2015.* https://www.europeristat.com/images/EPHR2015_web_hyperlinked_Euro-Peristat.pdf

Fagerberg, M. C., Marsal, K., & Kallen, K. (2015). Predicting the chance of vaginal delivery after one cesarean section: Validation and elaboration of a published prediction model. *European Journal of Obstetrics, Gynecology, & Reproductive Biology, 188*, 88-94. https://doi.org/10.1016/j.ejogrb.2015.02.031

Fair, C. D., Crawford, A., Houpt, B., & Latham, V. (2020). "After having a waterbirth, I feel like it's the only way people should deliver babies": The decision making process of women who plan a waterbirth. *Midwifery, 82*, 102622. https://doi.org/10.1016/j.midw.2019.102622

Fannin, M. (2019). Labour pain, 'natal politics' and reproductive justice for black birth givers. *Body & Society, 25*(3), 22-48. https://doi.org/10.1177/1357034x19856429

Fitzpatrick, K. E., Kurinczuk, J. J., Bhattacharya, S., & Quigley, M. A. (2019). Planned mode of delivery after previous cesarean section and short-term maternal and perinatal outcomes: A population-based record linkage cohort study in Scotland. *PLoS Med, 16*(9), e1002913. https://doi.org/10.1371/journal.pmed.1002913

Fox, D., Coddington, R., & Scarf, V. (2021). Wanting to be 'with woman', not with machine: Midwives' experiences of caring for women being continuously monitored in labour. *Women & Birth, S1871-5192(21)00153-0.* https://doi.org/10.1016/j.wombi.2021.09.002

Fox, D. D., Maude, D. R., Coddington, D. R., Woodworth, M. R., Scarf, D. V., Watson, D. K., & Foureur, P. M. (2020). The use of continuous fetal monitoring technologies that enable mobility in labour for women with complex pregnancies: A survey of Australian and New Zealand hospitals. *Midwifery*, 102887. https://doi.org/10.1016/j.midw.2020.102887

Fox, N. S. (2020). Pregnancy outcomes in patients with prior uterine rupture or dehiscence: A 5-year update. *Obstet Gynecol, 135*(1), 211-212. https://doi.org/10.1097/AOG.0000000000003622

Fox, N. S., Gerber, R. S., Mourad, M., Saltzman, D. H., Klauser, C. K., Gupta, S., & Rebarber, A. (2014). Pregnancy outcomes in patients with prior uterine rupture or dehiscence. *Obstetrics & Gynecol, 123*(4), 785-789. https://doi.org/10.1097/AOG.0000000000000181

Frederick, A., Fry, T., & Clowtis, L. (2020). Intraoperative mother and baby skin-to-skin contact during cesarean birth: Systematic review. *MCN: American Journal of Maternal/Child Nursing, 45*(5), 296-305.

Freidan, B. (2021). *The feminine mystique: The classic that sparked a feminist revolution*. Thread.

Funston, L., & Herring, S. (2016). When will the stolen generations end? A qualitative critical exploration of contemporary 'child protection' practices in Aboriginal and Torres Strait Islander communities. *Sexual Abuse in Australia and New Zealand, 7*(1), 51-58. http://ezproxy.uws.edu.au/login?url=https://www.proquest.com/scholarly-journals/when-will-stolen-generations-end-qualitative/docview/1805769481/se-2?accountid=36155

Gamble, J., Creedy, D., Moyle, W., Webster, J., McAllister, M., & Dickson, P. (2005). Effectiveness of a counseling intervention after a traumatic childbirth: A randomized controlled trial. *Birth, 32*(1), 11-19. https://doi.org/10.1111/j.0730-7659.2005.00340.x

Ganer Herman, H., Kogan, Z., Bar, J., & Kovo, M. (2017). Trial of labor after cesarean delivery for pregnancies complicated by gestational diabetes mellitus. *Internation Journal of Gynaecology & Obstetrics, 138*(1), 84-88. https://doi.org/10.1002/ijgo.12164

Garcia-Acosta, J. M., San Juan-Valdivia, R. M., Fernandez-Martinez, A. D., Lorenzo-Rocha, N. D., & Castro-Peraza, M. E. (2019). Trans* pregnancy and lactation: A literature review from a nursing perspective. *International Journal of Environmental Research & Public Health, 17*(1), 44. https://doi.org/10.3390/ijerph17010044

Geia, L., Baird, K., Bail, K., Barclay, L., Bennett, J., Best, O. et al. (2020). A unified call to action from Australian nursing and midwifery leaders: Ensuring that Black lives matter. *Contemporary Nurse, 56*(4), 297-308. https://doi.org/10.1080/10376178.2020.1809107

Gilbert, S., Grobman, A., Landon, M. B., Spong, C. Y., Rouse, D. J., Leveno, K. J. et al. (2012). Elective repeat cesarean delivery compared with spontaneous trial of labour after a prior cesarean delivery: A propensity-score analysis. *American Journal of Obstetrics and gynecology, 206*(311), 1-9.

Grobman, L. Y., Landon, M., Spong, C., Leveno, K., Rouse, D., Varner, M. et al. (2007). Development of a nomogram for prediction of vaginal birth after cesarean delivery. *Obstetrics & Gynecology, 109*(4), 806-812.

Grobman, W. A., Sandoval, G., Rice, M. M., Bailit, J. L., Chauhan, S. P., Costantine, M. M. et al. (2021). Prediction of vaginal birth after cesarean delivery in term gestations: A calculator without race and ethnicity. *American Journal of Obstetrics & Gynecology, 225*(6), P664,E1-664.E7. https://doi.org/10.1016/j.ajog.2021.05.021

Guiliano, M., Closset, E., Therby, D., LeGoueff, F., Deruelle, P., & Subtil, D. (2014). Signs, symptoms and complications of complete and partial uterine ruptures during pregnancy and delivery. *European Journal of Obstetrics, Gynecology, & Reproductive Biology, 179C*, 130-134. https://doi.org/10.1016/j.ejogrb.2014.05.004

Hairston, A. H. (1996). The debate over twilight sleep: Women influencing their medicine. *Journal of Women's Health, 5*(5), 489-499.

Hardeman, R. R., & Kozhimannil, K. B. (2016). Motivations for entering the doula profession: Perspectives from women of color. *Journal of Midwifery & Women's Health, 61*(6), 773-780. https://doi.org/10.1111/jmwh.12497

Hayase, M., & Shimada, M. (2018). Effects of maternity yoga on the autonomic nervous system during pregnancy. *Journal of Obstetrics and Gynaecology Research, 44*(10), 1887-1895. https://doi.org/10.1111/jog.13729

Hodgson, Z. G., Comfort, L. R., & Albert, A. A. Y. (2020). Water birth and perinatal outcomes in British Columbia: A retrospective cohort study. *Journal of Obstetrics & Gynaecology Canada, 42*(2), 150-155. https://doi.org/10.1016/j.jogc.2019.07.007

Homer, C., Wilson, A., & Davis, D. (2020). Editorial: Words matter; language matters. *Women & Birth, 33*(2), 105-106. https://doi.org/10.1016/j.wombi.2020.02.003

Homer, C. S. E., Davis, D. L., Mollart, L., Turkmani, S., Smith, R. M., Bullard, M., Leiser, B., & Foureur, M. (2021). Midwifery continuity of care and vaginal birth after caesarean section: A randomised controlled trial. *Women & Birth*, 35(3), e294-e301. https://doi.org/10.1016/j.wombi.2021.05.010

Hooks, B. (2000). *Feminism is for everybody: Passionate politics*. Pluto Press.

ICM (International College of Midwives). (2017). *Definition of midwifery*. https://www.internationalmidwives.org/assets/files/definitions-files/2018/06/eng-definition_midwifery.pdf

Inglis, S. (2002). Accessing a debriefing service following birth. *British Journal of Midwifery, 10*(6), 368-371.

Iyengar, B. (2013). *The tree of yoga the definitive guide to yoga in everyday life*. HarperThorsons.

Jahdi, F., Sheikhan, F., Haghani, H., Sharifi, B., Ghaseminejad, A., Khodarahmian, M., & Rouhana, N. (2017). Yoga during pregnancy: The effects on labor pain and delivery outcomes (A randomized controlled trial). *Complementary Therapies in Clinical Practice, 27*, 1-4. https://doi.org/10.1016/j.ctcp.2016.12.002

Johnson, B., & Quinlan, M. M. (2015). Technical versus public spheres: A feminist analysis of women's rhetoric in the twilight sleep debates of 1914–1916. *Health Communication, 30*(11), 1076- 1088. https://doi.org/10.1080/10410236.2014.921269

Jordan, B. (1997). Authoritative knowledge and its construction. In R. Davis-Floyd & C. Sargent (Eds.), *Childbirth and authoritative knowledge: Cross-cultural perspectives.* University of California Press.

Karaian, L. (2013). Pregnant men: Repronormativity, critical trans theory and the re(conceive)ing of sex and pregnancy in law. *Social & Legal Studies, 22*(2), 211-230. https://doi.org/10.1177/0964663912474862

Keedle, H., Schmied, V., Burns, E., & Dahlen, H. (2018a). The design, development, and evaluation of a qualitative data collection application for pregnant women. *Journal of Nursing Scholarship, 50*(1), 47-55. https://doi.org/10.1111/jnu.12344 (Journal of Nursing Scholarship)

Keedle, H., Schmied, V., Burns, E., & Dahlen, H. (2018b). The journey from pain to power: A meta-ethnography on women's experiences of vaginal birth after caesarean. *Women & Birth, 31*(1), 69- 79.

Keedle, H., Schmied, V., Burns, E., & Dahlen, H. G. (2015). Women's reasons for, and experiences of, choosing a homebirth following a caesarean section. *BMC Pregnancy Childbirth, 15*(1), 206. https://doi.org/10.1186/s12884-015-0639-4

Keedle, H. (2015). *Women's reasons for and experiences of having a homebirth following a previous caesarean experience* Western Sydney University]. Sydney. http://hdl.handle.net/1959.7/uws:34598

Keedle, H., Peters, L., Schmied, V., Burns, E., Keedle, W., & Dahlen, H. G. (2020). Women's experiences of planning a vaginal birth after caesarean in different models of maternity care in Australia. *BMC Pregnancy Childbirth, 20*(1), 381. https://doi.org/10.1186/s12884-020-03075-8

Keedle, H., Schmied, V., Burns, E., & Dahlen, H. G. (2019). A narrative analysis of women's experiences of planning a vaginal birth after caesarean (VBAC) in Australia using critical feminist theory. *BMC Pregnancy Childbirth, 19*(1), 142. https://doi.org/10.1186/s12884-019-2297-4

Kendall-Tacket, K. (2014). Birth trauma: The causes and consequences of childbirth-related trauma and PTSD. In D. L. Barnes (Ed.), *Women's reproductive mental health across the lifespan*. Springer International Publishing.

Kikuchi, J., Ranjit, A., Jiang, W., Witkop, C., Hamlin, L., & Koehlmoos, T. P. (2020). Early childhood outcomes among infants born by vaginal birth after cesarean and repeat cesarean delivery in the military health system. *Military Medicine, 186*(11-12), 1124-1128. https://doi.org/10.1093/milmed/usaa536

Kildea, S., Gao, Y., Hickey, S., Kruske, S., Nelson, C., Blackman, R., Tracy, S., Hurst, C., Williamson, D., & Roe, Y. (2019). Reducing preterm birth amongst Aboriginal and Torres Strait Islander babies: A prospective cohort study, Brisbane, Australia. *EClinicalMedicine, 12*, 43-51. https://doi.org/10.1016/j.eclinm.2019.06.001

Kitzinger, S. (1992). Sheila Kitzinger's letter from England: Birth plans. *Birth, 19*(1), 36-37. https://doi.org/10.1111/j.1523- 536x.1992.tb00373.x

Kitzinger, S. (2015). *A passion for birth: My life: Anthropology, family and feminism*. Pinter & Martin Limited.

Kozhimannil, K. B., & Hardeman, R. R. (2016). Coverage for doula services: How state medicaid programs can address concerns about maternity care costs and quality. *Birth, 43*(2), 97-99. https://doi.org/10.1111/birt.12213

Kozhimannil, K. B., Hardeman, R. R., Alarid-Escudero, F., Vogelsang, C. A., Blauer-Peterson, C., & Howell, E. A. (2016). Modeling the cost-effectiveness of doula care associated with reductions in preterm birth and cesarean delivery. *Birth, 43*(1), 20-27. https://doi.org/10.1111/birt.12218

Kusaka, M., Matsuzaki, M., Shiraishi, M., & Haruna, M. (2016). Immediate stress reduction effects of yoga during pregnancy: One group pre–post test. *Women & Birth, 29*(5), e82-e88. https://doi.org/10.1016/j.wombi.2016.04.003

Kwee, A., Smink, M., Van Der Laar, R., & Bruinse, H. W. (2007). Outcome of subsequent delivery after a previous early preterm cesarean section. *Journal of Maternal-Fetal & Neonatal Medicine, 20*(1), 33-37. https://doi.org/10.1080/14767050601036527

Kwon, R., Kasper, K., London, S., & Haas, D. M. (2020). A systematic review: The effects of yoga on pregnancy. *European Journal of Obstetrics, Gynecology & Reproductive Biology, 250*, 171-177. https://doi.org/10.1016/j.ejogrb.2020.03.044

Lakra, P., Patil, B., Siwach, S., Upadhyay, M., Shivani, S., Sangwan, V., & Mahendru, R. (2020). A prospective study of a new prediction model of vaginal birth after cesarean section at a tertiary care centre. *Journal of Turkish Society of Obstetric and Gynecology, 17*(4), 278-284. https://doi.org/10.4274/tjod.galenos.2020.82205

Latendresse, G., Murphy, P. A., & Fullerton, J. T. (2005). A description of the management and outcomes of vaginal birth after cesarean birth in the homebirth setting. *Journal of Midwifery & Women's Health, 50*(5), 386-391.

Lawrence, A., Lewis, L., Hofmeyr, G. J., & Styles, C. (2013). Maternal positions and mobility during first stage labour. *Cochrane database of systematic reviews*(10):CD003934. https://doi.org/10.1002/14651858.CD003934.pub4 (Cochrane Database of Systematic Reviews)

Leap, N., & Hunter, B. (2016). *Supporting women for labour and birth: A thoughtful guide*. Routledge.

Levett, K., & Dahlen, H. G. (2019). Perspective: Childbirth education in Australia: Have we lost our way? *Women & Birth, 32*(4), 291-293. https://doi.org/10.1016/j.wombi.2018.05.007

Levett, K., Smith, C. A., Bensoussan, A., & Dahlen, H. G. (2016a). The complementary therapies for labour and birth study making sense of labour and birth – Experiences of women, partners and midwives of a complementary medicine antenatal education course. *Midwifery, 40*, 124-131. https://doi.org/10.1016/j.midw.2016.06.011

Levett, K. M., Smith, C. A., Bensoussan, A., & Dahlen, H. G. (2016b). Complementary therapies for labour and birth study: A randomised controlled trial of antenatal integrative medicine for pain management in labour. *BMJ Open, 6*(7), e010691. https://doi.org/10.1136/bmjopen-2015-010691

Low, P. (2020). *Overview of the autonomic nervous system*. MSD Manual. https://www.msdmanuals.com/en-au/home/brain,- spinal-cord,-and-nerve-disorders/autonomic-nervous- system-disorders/overview-of-the-autonomic-nervous- system#

Lyell, D. (2011). Adhesions and perioperative complications of repeat cesarean delivery. *American Journal of Obstetrics & Gynecology, Supplement to December 2011*, S11-S18.

MacIvor Thompson, L. (2019). The politics of female pain: women's citizenship, twilight sleep and the early birth control movement. *Medical Humanities, 45*(1), 67-74. https://doi.org/10.1136/medhum-2017-011419

Macones, G. A., Peipert, J., Nelson, D. B., Odibo, A., Stevens, E. J., Stamilio, D. M. et al. (2005). Maternal complications with vaginal birth after cesarean delivery: a multicenter study [Multicenter Study Research Support, N.I.H., Extramural Research Support, U.S. Gov't, P.H.S.]. *American Journal of Obstetrics & Gynecology, 193*(5), 1656-1662. https://doi.org/10.1016/j.ajog.2005.04.002

Markou, G. A., Muray, J. M., & Poncelet, C. (2017). Risk factors and symptoms associated with maternal and neonatal complications in women with uterine rupture. A 16 years multicentric experience. *European Journal of Obstetrics, Gynecology and Reproductive Biology, 217*, 126-130. https://doi.org/10.1016/j.ejogrb.2017.09.001

Martin, Hamilton, B., Oserman, M., Driscoll, A., & Drake, P. (2018). *Births: Final data for 2016* (1). National Vital Statistics Reports, Issue.

McGarry, A., Stenfert Kroese, B., & Cox, R. (2016). How do women with an intellectual disability experience the support of a doula during their pregnancy, childbirth and after the birth of their child? *Journal of Applied Research in Intellectual Disabilities, 29*(1), 21-33. https://doi.org/https://doi.org/10.1111/jar.12155

McKenna, J. A., & Symon, A. G. (2014). Water VBAC: Exploring a new frontier for women's autonomy [Research Support, Non-U.S. Gov't]. *Midwifery, 30*(1), e20-25. https://doi.org/10.1016/j.midw.2013.10.004

McLeish, J., & Redshaw, M. (2019). "Being the best person that they can be and the best mum": a qualitative study of community volunteer doula support for disadvantaged mothers before and after birth in England. *BMC Pregnancy Childbirth, 19*, 21. https://doi.org/10.1186/s12884-018-2170-x

Mei, J. Y., Havard, A. L., Mularz, A. J., Maykin, M. M., & Gaw, S. L. (2019). Impact of obesity class on trial of labor after cesarean success: Does pre-pregnancy or at-delivery obesity status matter? *Journal of Perinatology, 39*(8), 1042-1049. https://doi.org/10.1038/s41372-019-0386-x

Miller, M. W., & Baker, S. (2021). African American women's experiences with birth after a prior cesarean section. *Maternal & Child Health Journal*, 26, 806-813. https://doi.org/10.1007/s10995-021-03277-2

Modzelewski, J., Jakubiak-Proc, M., Materny, A., Sotniczuk, M., Kajdy, A., & Rabijewski, M. (2019). Safety and success rate of vaginal birth after two cesarean sections: Retrospective cohort study. *Ginekologia Polska, 90*(8), 444-451. https://doi.org/10.5603/GP.2019.0076 (Ginekologia polska)

Mooney, S. S., Hiscock, R., Clarke, I. D. A., & Craig, S. (2019). Estimating success of vaginal birth after caesarean section in a regional Australian population: Validation of a prediction model. *Australian & New Zealand Journal of Obstetrics & Gynaecology, 59*(1), 66-70. https://doi.org/10.1111/ajo.12809

Mu, Y., Li, X., Zhu, J., Liu, Z., Li, M., Deng, K., Deng, C., Li, Q., Kang, L., & Wang, Y. (2018). Prior caesarean section and likelihood of vaginal birth, 2012–2016, China. *Bulletin of the World Health Organization, 96*(8), 548.

Mulherin, K., Miller, Y. D., Barlow, F. K., Diedrichs, P. C., & Thompson, R. (2013). Weight stigma in maternity care: Women's experiences and care providers' attitudes. *BMC Pregnancy Childbirth, 13*(1), 19. https://doi.org/10.1186/1471-2393-13-19

NAABB. (2020). *Black birthing bill of rights*. https://thenaabb.org/

Nachescu, V. (2009). Radical feminism and the nation: History and space in the political imagination of second-wave feminism. *Journal for the Study of Radicalism, 3*(1), 29-59. http://www.jstor.org.ezproxy.uws.edu.au/stable/41887617

Newnham, E. C., Moran, P. S., Begley, C. M., Carroll, M., & Daly, D. (2020). Comparison of labour and birth outcomes between nulliparous women who used epidural analgesia in labour and those who did not: A prospective cohort study. *Women & Birth, 34*(5), e435-e441. https://doi.org/10.1016/j.wombi.2020.09.001

Oakley, A. (1993). *Essays on women, medicine and health.* Edinburgh University Press.

Pairman, S., Tracy, S., Dahlen, H. G., & Dixon, L.. (2019). *Midwifery: Preparation for practice* (4th edition). Elsevier Chatswood, NSW : Elsevier Australia.

Palmer, K. (2021). *Changing the equation: Researchers remove race from a calculator for childbirth.* Stat News.

Patterson, L. S., O'Connell, C. M., & Baskett, T. F. (2002). Maternal and perinatal morbidity associated with classic and inverted T cesarean incisions. *Obstetrics & Gynecology, 100*(4), 633-637.

Paul, B., Mollmann, C. J., Kielland-Kaisen, U., Schulze, S., Schaarschmidt, W., Bock, N. et al. (2020). Maternal and neonatal outcome after vaginal breech delivery at term after cesarean section - A prospective cohort study of the Frankfurt breech at term cohort (FRABAT). *European Journal of Obstetrics, Gynecology, & Reproductive Biology, 252*, 594-598. https://doi.org/10.1016/j.ejogrb.2020.04.030

Pinterics, N. (2001). Riding the feminist waves: in with the third? *Canadian Woman Studies, 21*(4). https://cws.journals.yorku.ca/index.php/cws/article/view/6899

Pont, S., Austin, K., Ibiebele, I., Torvaldsen, S., Patterson, J., & Ford, J. (2018). Blood transfusion following intended vaginal birth after cesarean versus elective repeat cesarean section in women with a prior primary cesarean: A population-based record linkage study. *Acta Obstetrica & Gynecologica Scandinavica, 98(3), 382-389.* https://doi.org/10.1111/aogs.13504

Raja, S. N., Carr, D. B., Cohen, M., Finnerup, N. B., Flor, H., Gibson, S., et al. (2020). The revised International Association for the Study of Pain definition of pain: Concepts, challenges, and compromises. *Pain, 161*(9), 1976-1982. https://doi.org/10.1097/j.pain.0000000000001939

Rietveld, A. L., Teunissen, P. W., Kazemier, B. M., & De Groot, C. J. M. (2017). Effect of interpregnancy interval on the success rate of trial of labor after cesarean. *Journal of Perinatology, 37*(11), 1192-1196. https://doi.org/10.1038/jp.2017.117

Rosenstein, M. G., Nijagal, M., Nakagawa, S., Gregorich, S. E., & Kuppermann, M. (2015). The association of expanded access to a collaborative midwifery and laborist model with cesarean delivery rates. *Obstetrics & Gynecology, 126*(4), 716-723. http:// doi: 10.1097/AOG.0000000000001032.

Ross, L., & Solinger, R. (2017). *Reproductive justice: An introduction* (Vol. 1). Univ of California Press.

Saban, A., Shoham-Vardi, I., Yohay, D., & Weintraub, A. Y. (2019). Peritoneal adhesions are an independent risk factor for peri- and post-partum infectious morbidity. *European Journal of Obstetrics, Gynecology and Reproductive Biology, 241*, 60- 65. https://doi.org/10.1016/j.ejogrb.2019.08.001

Sandall, J., Soltani, H., Gates, S., Shennan, A., & Devane, D. (2016). Midwife led continuity models versus other models of care for childbearing women. *Cochrane Database of Systematic Reviews, 2016*(4), 1-122. https://doi.org/10.1002/14651858.CD004667.pub5

Sandall, J., Tribe, R. M., Avery, L., Mola, G., Visser, G. H. A., Homer, C. S. E. et al. (2018). Short-term and long-term effects of caesarean section on the health of women and children. *The Lancet, 392*(10155), 1349-1357. https://doi.org/https://doi.org/10.1016/S0140-6736(18)31930-5 (The Lancet)

Secchi, D., Albéric, J., Gobillot, S., Ghenassia, A., Roustit, M., Chauleur, C., Hoffmann, P., & Raia-Barjat, T. (2021). Balloon catheter vs oxytocin alone for induction of labor in women with one previous cesarean section and an unfavorable cervix: Amulticenter, retrospective study. *Archives of Gynecology & Obstetrics*. https://doi.org/10.1007/s00404-021-06298-y

Shinar, S., Agrawal, S., Hasan, H., & Berger, H. (2019). Trial of labor versus elective repeat cesarean delivery in twin pregnancies after a previous cesarean delivery—A systematic review and meta analysis. *Birth, 46*(4), 550-559. https://doi.org/10.1111/birt.12434

Simpson, M., Schmied, V., Dickson, C., & Dahlen, H. G. (2018). Postnatal post-traumatic stress: An integrative review. *Women & Birth, 31*(5), 367-379. https://doi.org/10.1016/j.wombi.2017.12.003

Snyder, R. C. (2008). What Is third-wave feminism? A new directions essay. *Signs, 34*(1), 175-196. https://doi.org/10.1086/588436

Stamilio, D. M., Defranco, E., Pare, E., Odibo, A., Peipert, J., Allsworth, J., Stevens, E., & Macones, G. (2007). Short interpregnancy interval. *Obstetrics & Gynecology, 110*(5), 1075-1082.

Stevens, J. (2015). Maternal-assisted caesarean section. *Midwifery Matters, 33*(2), 12-13.

Stevens, J., Schmied, V., Burns, E., & Dahlen, H. G. (2018). Who owns the baby? A video ethnography of skin-to-skin contact after a caesarean section. *Women & Birth, 31*(6), 453-462. https://doi.org/10.1016/j.wombi.2018.02.005

Stevens, J., Schmied, V., Burns, E., & Dahlen, H. G. (2019). Skin-to-skin contact and what women want in the first hours after a caesarean section. *Midwifery, 74*, 140-146. https://doi.org/10.1016/j.midw.2019.03.020

Stevens, J. R. (2018). *Facilitators, barriers and implications of immediate skin-to-skin contact after caesarean section: An ethnographic study.* Western Sydney University (Australia)].

Stock, S. J., Ferguson, E., Duffy, A., Ford, I., Chalmers, J., & Norman, J. E. (2013). Outcomes of induction of labour in women with previous caesarean delivery: A retrospective cohort study using a population database [Research Support, Non-U.S. Gov't]. *PLoS One, 8*(4), e60404. https://doi.org/10.1371/journal.pone.0060404

Tahseen, S., & Griffiths, M. (2010). Vaginal birth after two caesarean sections (VBAC-2)-a systematic review with meta-analysis of success rate and adverse outcomes of VBAC-2 versus VBAC-1 and repeat (third) caesarean sections. *BJOG, 117*(1), 5-19. https://doi.org/10.1111/j.1471-0528.2009.02351.x

Takeya, A., Adachi, E., Takahashi, Y., Kondoh, E., Mandai, M., & Nakayama, T. (2020). Trial of labor after cesarean delivery (TOLAC) in Japan: Rates and complications. *Archives of Gynecology & Obstetrics, 301*(4), 995-1001. https://doi.org/10.1007/s00404-020-05492-8

Tangel, V., White, R. S., Nachamie, A. S., & Pick, J. S. (2019). Racial and ethnic disparities in maternal outcomes and the disadvantage of peripartum black women: A multistate analysis, 2007–2014. *American Journal of Perinatology, 36*(08), 835-848. https://doi.org/10.1055/s-0038-1675207

Thomas, M.-P., Ammann, G., Brazier, E., Noyes, P., & Maybank, A. (2017). Doula services within a healthy start program: Increasing access for an underserved population. *Maternal and Child Health Journal, 21*(S1), 59-64. https://doi.org/10.1007/s10995-017-2402-0

Thornton, P. (2018). Limitations of vaginal birth after cesarean success prediction. *Journal of Midwifery & Women's Health, 63*(1), 115-120.

Togioka, B., & Tonismae, T. (2021). *Uterine rupture*. StatPearls Publishing. https://www.ncbi.nlm.nih.gov/books/NBK559209/

United Nations Population Fund. (2021). *The state of the world's midwifery 2021*. https://www.unfpa.org/sowmy#:~:text=The%20State%20of%20the%20World's%20Midwifery%202021%20calls%20for%20a,lives%20and%20improves%20health%20systems!

Van Der Pijl, M. S. G., Hollander, M. H., Van Der Linden, T., Verweij, R., Holten, L., Kingma, E. et al. (2020). Left powerless: A qualitative social media content analysis of the Dutch #breakthesilence campaign on negative and traumatic experiences of labour and birth. *PLoS One, 15*(5), e0233114. https://doi.org/10.1371/journal.pone.0233114

Vandenberghe, G., Bloemenkamp, K., Berlage, S., Colmorn, L., Deneux Tharaux, C., Gissler, M. et al. (2019). The international network of obstetric survey systems study of uterine rupture: A descriptive multi country population based study. *BJOG: An International Journal of Obstetrics & Gynaecology, 126*(3), 370-381.

Varner, M. W., Thom, E., Spong, C. Y., Landon, M. B., Leveno, K. J., Rouse, D. J. et al. (2007). Trial of labor after one previous cesarean delivery for multifetal gestation. *Obstetrics & Gynecology, 110*(4), 814-819. https://doi.org/10.1097/01.AOG.0000280586.05350.9e

Vedam, S., Stoll, K., Martin, K., Rubashkin, N., Partridge, S., Thordarson, D. et al. (2017a). The Mother's Autonomy in Decision Making (MADM) scale: Patient-led development and psychometric testing of a new instrument to evaluate experience of maternity care. *PLoS One, 12*(2), e0171804. https://doi.org/10.1371/journal.pone.0171804

Vedam, S., Stoll, K., McRae, D. N., Korchinski, M., Velasquez, R., Wang, J. et al. (2019). Patient-led decision making: Measuring autonomy and respect in Canadian maternity care. *Patient Education & Counseling, 102*(3), 586-594. https://doi.org/10.1016/j.pec.2018.10.023

Vedam, S., Stoll, K., Rubashkin, N., Martin, K., Miller-Vedam, Z., Hayes-Klein, H. et al. (2017b). The Mothers on Respect (MOR) index: Measuring quality, safety, and human rights in childbirth. *SSM Population Health, 3*, 201-210. https://doi.org/10.1016/j.ssmph.2017.01.005

Voultsos, P., Zymvragou, C. E., Karakasi, M. V., & Pavlidis, P. (2021). A qualitative study examining transgender people's attitudes towards having a child to whom they are genetically related and pursuing fertility treatments in Greece. *BMC Public Health, 21*(1). https://doi.org/10.1186/s12889-021-10422-7

Vyas, D. A., Jones, D. S., Meadows, A. R., Diouf, K., Nour, N. M., & Schantz-Dunn, J. (2019). Challenging the use of race in the vaginal birth after cesarean section calculator. *Womens Health Issues, 29*(3), 201-204. https://doi.org/10.1016/j.whi.2019.04.007

Wasserman, J. B., Abraham, K., Massery, M., Chu, J., Farrow, A., & Marcoux, B. C. (2018). Soft tissue mobilization techniques are effective in treating chronic pain following cesarean section: A multicenter randomized clinical trial. *Journal of Women's Health & Physical Therapy, 42*(3), 111-119. https://doi.org/10.1097/jwh.0000000000000103

Watson, K., Mills, T. A., & Lavender, D. T. (2018). The use of telemetry in labour: Results of a national online survey of UK maternity units. *British Journal of Midwifery, 26*(1), 14-19. https://doi.org/10.12968/bjom.2018.26.1.14

Whitburn, L. Y., Jones, L. E., Davey, M.-A., & McDonald, S. (2019). The nature of labour pain: An updated review of the literature. *Women and Birth, 32*(1), 28-38. https://doi.org/10.1016/j.wombi.2018.03.004

WHO. (2009). *WHO recommended interventions for improving maternal and newborn health*. World Health Organization.

Wilson, E., Sivanesan, K., & Veerasingham, M. (2020). Rates of vaginal birth after caesarean section: What chance do obese women have? *Australia & New Zealand Journal of Obstetrics & Gynaecology, 60*(1), 88-92. https://doi.org/10.1111/ajo.13003

Wilson, M., Jones, J., Butler, T., Simpson, P., Gilles, M., Baldry, E., Levy, M., & Sullivan, E. (2017). Violence in the lives of incarcerated Aboriginal mothers in Western Australia. *SAGE Open, 7*(1), 215824401668681. https://doi.org/10.1177/2158244016686814

Womersley, K., Ripullone, K., & Hirst, J. E. (2021). Tackling inequality in maternal health: Beyond the postpartum. *Future of Healthcare Journal, 8*(1), 31-35. https://doi.org/10.7861/fhj.2020-0275

Yam, S. (2020). Visualizing birth stories from the margin: Toward a reproductive justice model of rhetorical analysis. *Rhetoric & Society Quarterly, 50*(1), 19-34. https://doi.org/10.1080/02773945.2019.1682182

Yao, R., Crimmins, S. D., Contag, S. A., Kopelman, J. N., & Goetzinger, K. R. (2019). Adverse perinatal outcomes associated with trial of labor after cesarean section at term in pregnancies complicated by maternal obesity. *Journal of Maternal- Fetal & Neonatal Medicine, 32*(8), 1256-1261. https://doi.org/10.1080/14767058.2017.1404023

Zhang, T., & Liu, C. (2016). Comparison between continuing midwifery care and standard maternity care in vaginal birth after cesarean [Article]. *Pakistan Journal of Medical Sciences, 32*(3), 711-714. https://doi.org/10.12669/pjms.323.9546

Zhang, Y., Lauche, R., Cramer, H., Munk, N., & Dennis, J. A. (2021). Increasing trend of yoga practice among U.S. adults from 2002 to 2017. *Journal of Alternative and Complementary Medicine, 27(9), 778-785*. https://doi.org/10.1089/acm.2020.0506

Made in the USA
Middletown, DE
06 August 2022

70499416R00137